Cambridge Elements ≡

Elements in High-Risk Pregnancy: Management Options
edited by
David James
University of Nottingham
Philip Steer
Imperial College London
Carl Weiner
Creighton University School of Medicine
Stephen Robson
Newcastle University

MULTIPLE PREGNANCY

Jack Hamer
Birmingham Women's and Children's NHS Foundation Trust

Jennifer Tamblyn
Leeds NHS Teaching Hospital Trust

James Castleman
Birmingham Women's and Children's NHS Foundation Trust

R. Katie Morris
Institute of Applied Health Research, University of Birmingham

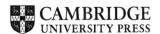

CAMBRIDGE
UNIVERSITY PRESS

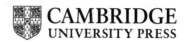

Shaftesbury Road, Cambridge CB2 8EA, United Kingdom

One Liberty Plaza, 20th Floor, New York, NY 10006, USA

477 Williamstown Road, Port Melbourne, VIC 3207, Australia

314–321, 3rd Floor, Plot 3, Splendor Forum, Jasola District Centre, New Delhi – 110025, India

103 Penang Road, #05–06/07, Visioncrest Commercial, Singapore 238467

Cambridge University Press is part of Cambridge University Press & Assessment, a department of the University of Cambridge.

We share the University's mission to contribute to society through the pursuit of education, learning and research at the highest international levels of excellence.

www.cambridge.org
Information on this title: www.cambridge.org/9781009526104

DOI: 10.1017/9781009526142

When citing this work, please include a reference to the DOI 10.1017/9781009526142

First published 2025

A catalogue record for this publication is available from the British Library

ISBN 978-1-009-52610-4 Paperback
ISSN 2976-8330 (online)
ISSN 2976-8322 (print)

Cambridge University Press & Assessment has no responsibility for the persistence or accuracy of URLs for external or third-party internet websites referred to in this publication and does not guarantee that any content on such websites is, or will remain, accurate or appropriate.

Every effort has been made in preparing this Element to provide accurate and up-to-date information which is in accord with accepted standards and practice at the time of publication. Although case histories are drawn from actual cases, every effort has been made to disguise the identities of the individuals involved. Nevertheless, the authors, editors and publishers can make no warranties that the information contained herein is totally free from error, not least because clinical standards are constantly changing through research and regulation. The authors, editors and publishers therefore disclaim all liability for direct or consequential damages resulting from the use of material contained in this Element. Readers are strongly advised to pay careful attention to information provided by the manufacturer of any drugs or equipment that they plan to use.

Multiple Pregnancy

Elements in High-Risk Pregnancy: Management Options

DOI: 10.1017/9781009526142
First published online: January 2025

Jack Hamer
Birmingham Women's and Children's NHS Foundation Trust

Jennifer Tamblyn
Leeds NHS Teaching Hospital Trust

James Castleman
Birmingham Women's and Children's NHS Foundation Trust

R. Katie Morris
Institute of Applied Health Research, University of Birmingham

Author for correspondence: R. Katie Morris, r.k.morris@bham.ac.uk

Abstract: Multiple pregnancy affects 0.9–3.1% of births worldwide. Prevalence rates vary significantly due to differences in dizygotic twinning rates and use of assisted reproduction. Both maternal and fetal/neonatal complications are more common in multiple compared to singleton pregnancies, and there are specific problems for the fetuses related to monochorionicity. Multiple pregnancies require specialised and individualised care. Complicated multiple pregnancies should be managed in a tertiary care centre where there is additional expertise, such as the laser ablation needed to treat monochorionic monozygotic pregnancies with conjoined circulations. Cornerstones of management in pregnancy are the need for accurate fetal measurement to optimise dating of gestational age, and documentation of chorionicity. High-level ultrasound expertise is needed. The mothers need frequent assessment to detect hypertension and anemia, and early identification and management of preterm labour.

Keywords: higher-order multiples, monochorionic, multiple pregnancy, selective fetal growth restriction, twin-to-twin transfusion syndrome

ISBNs: 9781009526104 (PB), 9781009526142 (OC)
ISSNs: 2976-8330 (online), 2976-8322 (print)

Contents

Commentary

Multiple pregnancy affects 0.9–3.1% of births worldwide. Prevalence rates vary significantly. For example, twinning rates are 6–9 per 1,000 births in East Asia, but 18 per 1,000 in central Africa. This variation is due to differences in dizygotic (DZ; non-identical) twinning rates (thought to be genetic). Monozygotic (MZ; identical) twinning occurs at a relatively constant rate of 3.5–4 per 1,000 around the globe. In high-income countries, there is further variation related to the use of assisted reproduction (AR). For example, in England and Wales, 14.4 out of every 1,000 women giving birth in 2020 had a multiple birth, whereas in the United States, the twin rate was 31.1 per 1,000 live births, and triplet and higher-order births comprised 79.6 per 100,000 births. Because of the higher morbidity and mortality of twin pregnancies, in recent years there has been a concerted effort to restrict AR to single embryo transfer (SET), which is associated with a significantly lower rate of multiple pregnancy compared to transferring more than one embryo. For example, in the UK in 2006, the Human Fertilisation and Embryology Authority (HFEA) published a report with a set of policies in order to reduce multiple births from AR, including SET. Single embryo transfers increased from 13% of in vitro fertilisation (IVF) cycles in 1991 to 75% in 2019, and a reduction in the multiple birth rate was seen from 27% in 2007 to 6% in 2019 in patients aged 35 and under.

Both maternal and fetal/neonatal complications are more common in multiple compared to singleton pregnancies. The main maternal problems during pregnancy include anemia, hypertensive disorders, gestational diabetes, haemorrhage and intrahepatic cholestasis of pregnancy (ICP). Preterm labour and caesarean section are commoner than in a singleton pregnancy. Fetal problems common to all multiple births include congenital abnormalities, miscarriage, single fetal death, growth disorders and cerebral palsy. Chorionicity (the number of chorions/placentas) and zygosity (the degree of genetic similarity/dissimilarity) affect these risks. Thus, some complications such as conjoined twins and monoamniotic (MA) twins only occur in monochorionic (MC) MZ pregnancies because they result from an abnormal connection between the two circulations in a shared placenta. In DZ twins, each twin has its own separate placenta and circulation, even though they may be adjacent.

Multiple pregnancies require specialised and individualised care. Usually, this is provided by a multidisciplinary team comprising an experienced midwife and obstetrician, allowing discussion and decision-making, and access to immediate diagnostic ultrasound (US) and multidisciplinary opinions such as anaesthetic, neonatal/paediatric and psychological services. Complicated multiple pregnancies should be managed in a tertiary care centre where there is add-itional expertise, such as the laser ablation needed to treat MCMZ pregnancies with conjoined circulations.

Cornerstones of management in pregnancy are the need for accurate fetal measurement to optimise dating of gestational age, and documentation of chorionicity. High-level US expertise is needed because of the high incidence of fetal anomaly, the need for detailed evaluation of the fetal circulations and the difficulty of assessing fetal size (and growth) in a 'crowded' uterus. The mothers need frequent assessment to detect hypertension and anemia, and early identification and management of preterm labour.

Delivery should take place in an obstetric unit with level 3 neonatal care, both because of the high incidence of preterm birth (average gestational length is only 36 weeks in twins and 34 weeks in triplets) and the high incidence of hypoxic and mechanical complications of labour. An experienced obstetrician, midwife and anaesthetist must be available 24/7. A neonatal paediatrician and a neonatal team should be available for delivery, with one paediatrician present for each infant, especially if preterm or operative delivery or fetal abnormalities are anticipated. The timing of delivery is determined by chorionicity and the presence of complications. The mode of delivery is influenced by the fetal presentations, the difference in birthweights (BWs), gestational age, the pres-ence of fetal complications and the woman's preferences. Active management of the third stage of labour is advocated. After delivery, the mother will need extra support both in hospital and at home.

1 Introduction

'Multiple pregnancy' is a pregnancy with two or more fetuses, including twins (the commonest multifetal pregnancy), triplets and higher-order multiples. The overall prevalence of multiple pregnancy varies worldwide from 0.9 to 3.1% [1,2,3,4]. The rate of MZ twin (identical twins) birth rate remains fairly constant at a rate of 3.5–4.0 per 1,000 around the globe [4]. Thus, the variation across different populations is due to variation in DZ births; this is thought to mainly be influenced by genetics and is reflected in racial and ethnic differences, with low rates of 1.3 per 1,000 births in Japan and rates as high as 50 per 1,000 births in Nigeria [5]. Substantial increases in twinning rates have been observed in Europe, North America and Asia. Africa is the continent with the highest rates at 17.1 per 1,000 deliveries, and Asia is the lowest at 9.2 per 1,000. Due to population growth, Asia and Africa are now home to more than 80% of the world's twin births [4,6]. A shift towards an older maternal age at conception has also contributed to the increasing rates [7]. In high-income countries, there is further variation related to the use of AR. For example, in 2021, 13.7 per 1,000 women giving birth in England and Wales had a multiple birth, whereas in the United States, the twin birth rate was 31.2 per 1,000 live births [1,2].

Until recently, the incidence of multiple births within England and Wales was continually rising, reflecting the effects of increased maternal age, parity and use of AR. Following the introduction of ovulation induction and multiple-embryo-transfer fertility, the UK triplet rate more than quadrupled between 1970 and 1998. However, since 1998, triplet and higher-order multiple rates have fallen annually, most likely reflecting changes in AR practice and guidance. In 2006, the HFEA published a report entitled 'One Child at a Time' with a set of policies to reduce multiple births from AR, including SET [8]. Single embryo transfers were seen to increase from 13% of IVF cycles in 1991 to 75% in 2019, and a reduction in the multiple birth rate was seen from 27% in 2007 to 6% in 2019 in patients aged 35 and under [9]. Office for National Statistics (ONS) data from 2021 for England and Wales demonstrated that twin pregnancy rates have continued to decrease, with birth rates equivalent to reported rates in 1996 [1]. In England and Wales in 2021, only 102 women gave birth to triplets and there was one higher-order multiple pregnancy (live born or stillborn) [1]. Multiple birth rates have also been affected by the use of selective reduction (SR; often in the first trimester).

1.1 Developmental Aspects

Multiple pregnancies are either polyzygotic (PZ) or MZ. Dizygotic twins are far more common than MZ twins, accounting for approximately 70% of all twin pregnancies [5]. In PZ pregnancies, each embryo is derived from a different ovum and, thus, are 'non-identical'. This arises when polyovulation occurs in a cycle, with dual fertilisation from a single source. Each zygote will develop its own amnion, chorion and placental circulation and can be defined as 'polychorionic'.

In MZ pregnancies, a zygote is formed from the union of one ovum and one sperm, which subsequently divides to form two 'identical' individuals (Figure 1) [10], although this is not invariable as both genotypic and phenotypic differences can sometimes occur. The pattern of placentation is dependent primarily upon the timing of division. In general, when division occurs within three days of fertilisation, dichorionic (DC) placentation occurs, in which each fetus has its own placental circulation. Division at three to nine days results in MC twin placentation, in which there is sharing of one placenta. Similarly, amnionicity, which reflects the number of gestational sacs present, is largely dependent upon the timing of division. Splitting after nine days results in MA

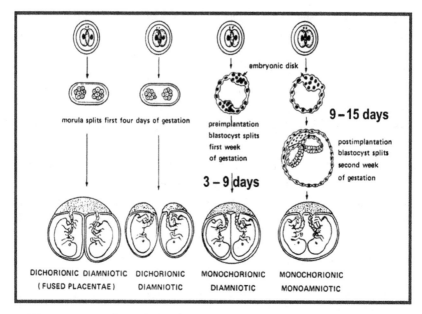

Figure 1 MZ twins: relationship between chorionicity and amnionicity. Reproduced with permission from Ward, RH, Whittle, MJ (eds). Multiple Pregnancy. London: RCOG Press, 1995

twins, in which one sac is shared by both [11]. Before this, each fetus forms and develops an individual sac. Monoamnionicity is rare, representing <1% of twin pregnancies [11]. Cleavage occurring after the 12th day will result in conjoined twins. For triplet and higher-order multiples the same principles apply, with different combinations of chorionicity and amnionicity possible (e.g., DC triamniotic (DCTA) triplets would comprise an MC diamniotic (MCDA) twin pair and a 'singleton'). From a clinical perspective, it is chronicity that influences pregnancy risk and management.

2 Risks Related to Multiple Pregnancies

2.1 Maternal Risks

Women with a multiple pregnancy are at an increased risk of obstetric complications, severe maternal morbidity and mortality. Table 1 shows that many maternal conditions are more likely in a multifetal pregnancy. Women with multiple pregnancies are also more prone to minor complications of pregnancy, including increased abdominal pain, malaise, acid reflux, poor sleep, constipation, varicose veins, dependent oedema and symphysiopubic dysfunction. These women therefore require more frequent monitoring than those with low-risk singleton pregnancies.

Table 1 Maternal risks associated with multiple pregnancy with associated singleton and multiple gestation prevalence

Maternal risks	Singleton pregnancy prevalence (%)	Multiple pregnancy prevalence (%)
Hyperemesis gravidarum (Section 2.1.1)	1.3	2.9 [15]
Anemia (Section 2.1.2)	38.7	67.3 [16]
Urinary tract infections (Section 2.1.3)	19.0	17.0 [17]
Hypertension and pre-eclampsia/eclampsia (Section 2.1.4)	6.5	12.7–20.0 [18,19,20]
Gestational diabetes (Section 2.1.5)	4.8	6.8 [21]
ICP and other liver disease (Section 2.1.6)	1.3	6.7 [22]
Haemorrhage (>1,000 ml) (Section 2.1.7)	8.7	17.0 [23,24]
Idiopathic polyhydramnios (Section 2.1.8)	0.4–3.3	0.4–3.3[*] [25]
Preterm labour/birth (Section 2.1.9)	8.2	60.3 [26]
Operative vaginal birth (Section 2.1.10)	5.3	14.0 [27,28]
Caesarean section (Section 2.1.11)	23.8	42.9 [29,30]
Postnatal illness (Section 2.1.12)	8.3	11.3 [31]
Maternal morbidity and mortality (Section 2.1.13)	1.3 / 0.1	6.2 [32] / 0.4 [14]

*An increased incidence of polyhydramnios in multiple pregnancy can be seen due to complications of monochorionicity and/or the presence of fetal anomalies. There is no evidence that uncomplicated multiple pregnancy has an increased risk of idiopathic polyhydramnios.

Twin pregnancy is associated with greater severe maternal morbidity and mortality [12,13]. Maternal mortality is also higher than in singleton pregnancy [14].

For many of these risks the management will be the same as for singleton pregnancy. Those where management may vary in multiple pregnancy will be discussed further in Section 3.

2.1.1 Hyperemesis Gravidarum

Nausea and vomiting are common and seen in approximately 50–90% of pregnant women [33], and multiple pregnancy is a known risk factor for worsening symptoms. The most severe form, hyperemesis gravidarum, has been shown in systematic reviews to occur in 0.3–10.8% of pregnancies [34]. A UK population study demonstrated a prevalence of 1.48% and an increased risk in twins compared to singletons, adjusted odds ratio (AOR: 2.09, 95% confidence interval (CI): 2.02–2.16) [35]. This is similar to another large cohort that demonstrated a 61% increase in the development of hyperemesis gravidarum in twin pregnancies compared to singletons [36]. In any woman diagnosed with hyperemesis gravidarum, a first-trimester US should be performed to diagnose or exclude a multiple pregnancy.

2.1.2 Anemia

Secondary to increased oxygen demands and plasma volume expansion (one-third greater than singletons), the risk of anemia is heightened in multiple pregnancy. A study of 2,130 pregnancies (1,684 singletons and 446 twin pregnancies) revealed 67.3% of twin pregnancies were anemic (defined as Hb <105 g/l) compared with 38.7% of singleton pregnancies [16]. Fetal demands are also greater, particularly for folate.

2.1.3 Urinary Tract Infections

Urinary tract infections are more common in twin and triplet pregnancies than in singleton pregnancies [17]. The incidence of pyelonephritis does not appear to be increased [37].

2.1.4 Hypertensive Disorders

Gestational hypertension and/or pre-eclampsia complicate 10–20% of multiple pregnancies, which is an incidence of two- to five-times higher than in singleton pregnancies [20,38]. However, it is likely the true underlying tendency is underestimated, as many multiple gestations will deliver preterm compared to singleton pregnancies, so birth occurs before worsening hypertensive disease ensues. There are many different pathophysiological processes that may contribute to the increased risk, which appears to be dose-dependent (i.e., reliant on placental mass and number of fetuses), with reported rates in triplets of 20.0% compared to 12.7% in twins [39]. The incidence is also higher among nulliparous compared to parous women. Importantly, the onset, progression and severity of pre-eclampsia are often sooner, quicker and greater in multiple pregnancies [37,40].

As such, this results in higher rates of eclampsia, placental abruption and maternal mortality and neonatal adverse outcomes [41,42].

2.1.5 Gestational Diabetes

Women with multiple pregnancies may also be at increased risk of gestational diabetes [16]. A study of 759,718 singleton and twin deliveries published in 2021 highlighted a prevalence of gestational diabetes in twins at 6.82% compared to 4.8% in singletons [16]. A dose–response relationship exists with higher rates in higher-order multiples [41].

2.1.6 ICP and Other Liver Disease

The incidence of ICP in multiple pregnancy is higher, with some studies reporting rates of up to 22% [37,43]. Data published in 2018 reported that twin pregnancies conceived through AR are twice as likely to develop ICP compared with spontaneously conceived twin pregnancies [44]. A retrospective cohort study demonstrated rates of ICP of 6.7% in twins versus 1.3% in singletons [22]. An increased risk of adverse outcome has also been reported associated with total bile acid levels [22]. Twin pregnancy is also an independent risk factor for acute fatty liver, a rare complication of pregnancy associated with significant maternal mortality [37].

2.1.7 Haemorrhage

There is a high incidence of antepartum and postpartum haemorrhage (PPH), with the average blood loss 500 ml higher than in a singleton pregnancy [24,37]. Antepartum bleeding is particularly common. A major cause is placental abruption, which may arise secondary to uterine over distension and decompression following rupture of membranes or first twin delivery [37]. The larger placental surface area in multiple pregnancy is also considered a predisposing factor for placenta praevia [45], and the incidence of velamentous cord insertion and vasa previa is also increased [37,46]. Increased placental surface area, uterine over distension and higher caesarean section rates all contribute to the increased risk of postpartum blood loss. Other characteristics associated with PPH >1,000 ml in twins include episiotomy and neonatal weight [23].

2.1.8 Polyhydramnios

Multiple pregnancies account for about 10% of cases of polyhydramnios [47]. This may be idiopathic, related to gestational complications such as maternal diabetes, or relate to specific complications of monochorionicity such as twin-to-twin transfusion syndrome (TTTS) [37]. In this setting, the risks of preterm labour and/ or preterm rupture of membranes, cord prolapse, malpresentation and abdominal discomfort are increased [47].

2.1.9 PTB

Approximately 50% of all multiple pregnancies birth preterm (<37 complete weeks' gestation), and they account for about 20% of all preterm births (PTBs) [26,48,49]. Large variation in PTB rates has been reported. In Scotland (n = 1,432 live multiple births), 9.9% delivered before 32 weeks, 41.3% at 32–6 weeks and 51.2% before 37 weeks, whereas in Austria (n = 2,311), 12.7% delivered before 32 weeks, 55.7% at 32–6 weeks and 68.4% before 37 weeks [50]. The rate of PTB is significantly increased in MC compared to DC twins, likely to be related to the complications of monochorionicity [51]. Risks to the mother relate to the need for hospitalisation, use of tocolytics and possible intrauterine transfer.

2.1.10 Operative Vaginal Birth

Compared to singleton pregnancies, there is an increased rate of operative vaginal births [27,28]. The maternal risks associated with instrumental delivery are the same as for singleton birth.

2.1.11 Caesarean Section

Women with multiple pregnancy are more likely to have an elective or emergency caesarean section, with rates as high as 75% reported worldwide [52]. A 2019 Cochrane review reported that 42.9% of women with multiple pregnancy who aimed for a vaginal birth had a caesarean section for at least one fetus [29].

2.1.12 Postnatal Illness

A 2011 systematic review concluded that multiple birth might be associated with an increased risk of postpartum depressive symptoms [53]. Given the high fetal morbidity and mortality rates associated with multiple pregnancy, bereavement and grief support are often required. Furthermore, with the potential psychosocial and financial difficulties associated with multiple pregnancy, a high index of suspicion for postnatal depression is recommended [53].

2.1.13 Maternal Morbidity and Mortality

Severe maternal morbidity is increased in multiple pregnancy [12], with comparative studies demonstrating that the relative risk (RR) of severe maternal morbidity compared to singletons was 4.3 (95% CI: 3.7–5.0). Risks were higher in triplets (RR: 6.2, 95% CI: 2.5–15.3) [13].

Maternal mortality is 2.5-times higher in multiple than in singleton births in the UK [54] and World Health Organisation (WHO) multi-country survey data demonstrated rates of maternal death of 0.4% in twins and 0.1% in singletons [14]. Specific factors contributing to maternal death in multiple births are the use of tocolytic agents, pre-eclampsia and eclampsia, placental abruption, caesarean delivery and PPH [37].

2.2 Fetal Risks

Women with multiple pregnancy are also at increased risk of fetal complications, as shown in Table 2.

Table 2 Fetal risks associated with multiple pregnancy with associated singleton and multiple gestation prevalence

Fetal risks	Singleton pregnancy prevalence (%)	Multiple pregnancy prevalence (%)
Congenital anomalies (Section 2.2.1)	2.70	3.49 [3]
Structural	2.35	3.23
Chromosomal	0.35	0.26
Early pregnancy loss (Section 2.2.2)	5.40*	15.00–35.00 [55,56]
Single fetal death (Section 2.2.3)	0.40	6.00 [57,58]
Discordant fetal growth and growth restriction (Section 2.2.4)	8.00	25.00 [59]
Preterm birth (Section 2.2.5)	8.20	60.30 [2]
Cord prolapse (Section 2.2.6)	0.10–0.60	Up to 1.80 [60,61]
Twin entrapment (Section 2.2.7)	N/A	0.10 [62]
Cerebral palsy (Section 2.2.8)	0.20	0.70–5.10 [63,64]
Perinatal mortality^ (Section 2.2.9)	0.14–0.32	0.62–0.73 [65]

* Overall figure for pregnancy loss <20 weeks after confirmation of fetal heart activity, but ranges from 0.8 to 33.7% based on gestational age and number of prior pregnancy losses [55]

^ Range given as perinatal mortality rate depends on chorionicity

2.2.1 Congenital Anomalies

There is an increased risk of congenital anomalies in multiple pregnancy compared to singletons, reported as 27% higher [66]. In Europe, the prevalence has increased from 5.9 per 10,000 multiple births in 1984–7 to 10.7 per 10,000 in 2004–7. Non-chromosomal anomalies increased from 5.03 per 10,000 births to 10.00 over the same period, it is suggested that this may relate to an increased risk in DC twins conceived by AR or to parental characteristics associated with AR. For chromosomal anomalies, the prevalence increased from 0.58 per 10,000 births to 0.90 [3].

The risk rate per fetus for DZ twins is most likely similar to that of singletons, but two- to three-times higher in MZ twins, which reflects primarily an increased risk of abnormal cleavage and midline structural defects, including syringomyelia, cloacal anomalies and holoprosencephaly [66,67,68].

Approximately 1 in 25 DC, 1 in 15 MCDA and 1 in 6 MA twin pregnancies are discordant for anomaly, with a major structural defect affecting only one fetus [68,69]. The European data recorded that for twin pairs with at least one non-chromosomal abnormality, there was concordance in 11.6% [3]. The most common structural defects in twin pregnancies include cardiac anomalies, neural tube defects, brain defects, facial clefts, and gastrointestinal and anterior abdominal wall defects [70]. A 2020 study of 488 twins reported the rates of different structural anomalies: genitourinary defects represented 24%, with cardiac and gastrointestinal anomalies representing 20 and 18.5%, respectively [71]. Importantly, if a discordant anomaly is noted, the likelihood is that it will originate within the smaller twin, however, the risk of adverse outcome for the normal twin is also increased [71,72].

Monozygotic twins are generally concordant for chromosomal or genetic defects (although discordance may occur secondary to postzygotic mutation, parental imprinting effects, asymmetrical X inactivation and differential deoxyribonucleic acid (DNA) methylation) [10]. European data report that for chromosomal anomalies, 5.53% of all twin pairs were concordant [3]. For DZ pregnancies, the risk of chromosomal abnormalities for each twin is no different to that for a singleton fetus, but since two fetuses are present, the chance of one being affected is doubled. For MZ pregnancies, the baseline risk is twice that of a singleton pregnancy, therefore four-times higher for at least one twin to be affected [73,74].

The implications of AR for DZ twin congenital anomaly rates are not fully understood, but recent data have demonstrated an increased risk of congenital heart defects in twin pregnancies conceived with AR compared to spontaneously conceived pregnancies [75].

There are also congenital anomalies that are considered unique to twin pregnancies [55]:

- midline structural defects, believed to be a consequence of the twinning process (e.g., conjoined twins)
- malformations resulting from vascular events as a consequence of placental anastomoses. Following co-twin demise, the following can occur: microcephaly, periventricular leukomalacia, hydrocephalus, intestinal atresia, renal dysplasia or limb amputation
- defects or deformities from intrauterine 'crowding': foot deformities, hip dislocation and skull asymmetry

The spectrum of abnormalities specific to MZ twins are categorised either as 'symmetrical' (namely, conjoined twins) or 'asymmetrical' duplications. The latter are further subdivided into those with a separate external twin present (twin reversed arterial perfusion (TRAP) sequence), an attached fetal mass (ectoparasitic twins) or an internal asymmetrical duplication (endoparasitic twins or fetus-in-fetu) [10].

2.2.2 Early Pregnancy Loss

Mortality of one or more fetuses within the first trimester is a common occurrence with a reported prevalence of between 15 and 35%. However, the mortality rate can be up to 50% in pregnancies that began with three or more gestational sacs [56,76]. The true prevalence of fetal loss is likely to be even greater, as many twin pregnancies are initially undetected if not monitored with sequential sonographic evaluation during the first trimester. The so-called vanishing twin syndrome (VTS) occurs when a late first-trimester scan identifies fewer fetuses than an earlier scan. Several aetiologies have been proposed, including chromosomal abnormalities, placental 'crowding', chronic maternal disease and inappropriate implantation [56].

Vanishing twin syndrome is identified more frequently in AR pregnancies, mostly because of the increased prevalence of multiple pregnancy with AR, but in addition, due to the increased frequency of early pregnancy scanning in AR pregnancies. The number of embryos initially transferred has also been shown to increase the occurrence of VTS [77]. Within the context of AR and double embryo transfer (DET), the vanishing twin phenomenon is associated with an increased risk of PTB and low BW (LBW) in both fresh and frozen embryo cycles when multiple gestational sacs were initially visualised [78]. In other settings, the impact on the surviving co-twin is not known to be adverse, although data remain sparse.

Fetus papyraceous occurs when one twin dies at an early gestation and becomes shrunken and compressed.

A 10-year multicentre retrospective study including 3,117 twin pregnancies (605 MC and 2,512 DC) concluded that the risk of early pregnancy loss before 24 weeks was significantly higher in MC twins (60.3 per 1,000 fetuses) than in DC twins (6.6 per 1,000 fetuses), with an RR of 9.18. The study also demonstrated that the rate of fetal loss in MC pregnancies was highest at 16–22 weeks' gestation, likely due to the corresponding peak in incidence of TTTS [79]. Early detection of MC pregnancies is therefore paramount. The risk of subsequent miscarriage in twin pregnancies with one missed early silent miscarriage of one fetus is also increased: it is approximately 10-times higher than in twin pregnancies unaffected by single miscarriage [80].

2.2.3 Single Fetal Death

Single twin demise (>14 weeks' gestation) occurs in approximately 5–6% of twin pregnancies and may occur in any trimester [58]. The risk of single intrauterine fetal demise (sIUFD) is seen to be greater with MC (7.5%) than DC (3%) twins, likely due to inter-twin placental anastomoses causing an adverse distribution of placental blood flow [58,81]. The etiology of fetal demise may be either fetal (infection, chromosomal or structural anomaly), cord incident or placental (TTTS or selective fetal growth restriction (sFGR)), or maternal (hypertensive disorders, thrombophilia, abruption). A UK population study of 81 MC twin pregnancies with sIUFD published in 2020 identified that 47% were due to TTTS [81].

Fetal morbidity and mortality are both increased in the remaining co-twin, due either to the potential risk from the same pathophysiological condition that affected the sibling or to the death of the sibling. There are two main theories to explain the risk of morbidity and mortality for the co-twin: transient hemodynamic fluctuations and transchorionic embolisation. Systematic reviews and meta-analysis identified that the rates of co-twin demise were 15% (95% CI: 9.1–20.9) for MC twins and 3% (95% CI: 0.4–5.7) for DC twins (odds ratio (OR): 5.24, 95% CI: 1.75–15.7) with an increased risk of co-twin demise in MC pregnancies if the fetal death occurred prior to 28 weeks [58,82]. For the surviving twin, the subsequent risks were profoundly increased, particularly in an MC pregnancy. Specifically, the risk of PTB was increased due to iatrogenic deliveries at 60.4% (95% CI: 33.5–109.1) in MC twins, compared with 32.7% (95% CI: 14.6–72.1) in DC pregnancies, respectively [58]. The risk of neurological abnormality, including cerebral palsy, in the surviving co-twin was 20% (95% CI: 12.8–31.1) for MC twins, with prior literature demonstrating a risk of just 2% (95% CI: 1.6–4.9) for DC twins [58,82]. Large prospective multicentre studies with shared protocols for prenatal management are warranted, particularly looking at neurodevelopmental comorbidity in the surviving twin.

2.2.4 Discordant Fetal Growth and Fetal Growth Restriction

The growth of twins does not differ significantly from singleton growth in the first and second trimesters. However, from 32 weeks' gestation, slower fetal growth is often observed. If singleton growth charts are used, growth 'abnormalities' in twins are overestimated compared with the use of twin growth charts, as the definition of small for gestational age (SGA) remains the same, an estimated fetal weight (EFW) <10th centile [83,84]. However, it is possible that the usual slower growth of twins in the third trimester may reflect a state of 'relative growth restriction' compared with singleton gestations [85]. A certain degree of weight discordance (~10%) between twins is generally recognised as a normal physiological variation, greater discordance is seen as an independent risk factor for adverse perinatal outcomes regardless of chorionicity [86].

Fetal growth is determined by several factors including genetic differences in growth potential (DC twins), unequal uteroplacental perfusion to each twin, congenital infection affecting one fetus or aberrant placental umbilical cord insertion [84,87,88]. Relevant maternal factors increasing the risk of suboptimal fetal growth in multiple pregnancies include older age, nulliparity, assisted conception and gestational hypertension.

Fetal growth restriction (FGR) is more common in multiple pregnancies, with around 25% of twin pregnancies affected, and in each individual fetus the definition for FGR is the same as in singletons, as is the definition of SGA. However, in twins, the difference in growth between the two fetuses (discordance) also needs to be considered as this is associated with greater perinatal risks [86]. A Delphi consensus definition of FGR and sFGR (see Section 2.3) has been proposed [89].

To calculate the discordance in growth, the following equation is used, using EFW in utero or BW:

[(Larger estimated or actual weight – smaller estimated or actual weight)/ larger estimated or actual weight] × 100

Several thresholds for significant discordance have been suggested with the commonest reported in the literature ranging between 18 and 30% [90]. The prospective ESPRIT (Evaluation of Sonographic Predictors of Restricted Growth in Twins) study concluded that the threshold for significant growth discordance, defined according to adverse perinatal outcome risk, should be 18% for both DC and MC twins without TTTS. In the setting of MC with TTTS, this cut-off was lowered to 15% [91]. A 2018 review of 10,877 twin pregnancies reported that in DC pregnancies, there was found to be a greater risk of intrauterine death (IUD), but not neonatal death (NND) in twins with a BW discordance of 15% (OR: 9.8, 95% CI: 3.9–29.4), $\geq$ 20% (OR: 7.0, 95% CI: 4.15–11.8), $\geq$25% (OR: 17.4, 95% CI: 8.3–36.7) and $\geq$30% (OR: 22.9, 95% CI: 10.2–51.6), respectively, compared with those without BW discordance [90]. Within each cut-off of BW discordance, the smaller twin was at a greater risk of mortality compared with the larger one. In MC twin gestations, excluding cases affected by TTTS, twins with BW discordance $\geq$20% (OR: 2.8, 95% CI: 1.3–5.8) or $\geq$25% (OR: 3.2, 95% CI: 1.5–6.7) were at higher risk of IUD, compared with controls [92]. The overall risk of mortality in MC pregnancies was similar between the smaller and larger twin, except in those with BW discordance $\geq$20% [90].

The Royal College of Obstetricians and Gynaecologists (RCOG), the International Society of Ultrasound in Obstetrics and Gynecology (ISUOG) and the American College of Obstetricians and Gynecologists (ACOG) all report that a cut-off of 20% should be adopted, whilst the Fetal Medicine Foundation (FMF) recognise a $\geq$25% discordance between the two fetuses as selective growth restriction [93,94,95].

Discordance in fetal growth is an independent risk factor for neonatal morbidity. A 2019 study conducted by di Mascio et al. demonstrated that the risk of composite morbidity was significantly higher in the pregnancies with BW discordance $\geq$15% (OR: 1.4, 95% CI: 1.0–1.9), $\geq$20% (OR: 2.2, 95% CI: 1.40–3.45), $\geq$25% (OR: 2.5, 95% CI: 1.8–3.6) and $\geq$30% (OR: 3.4, 95% CI: 2.2–3.2) [96]. In DC, BW discordance $\geq$15% (OR: 2.4, 95% CI: 1.65–3.46), $\geq$20% (OR: 2.2, 95% CI: 1.3–3.8), $\geq$25% (OR: 2.7, 95% CI: 1.4–5.1) and $\geq$30% (OR: 3.6, 95% CI: 2.3–5.7) were all significantly associated with composite neonatal morbidity [96].

Given the significant association between twin weight difference and adverse perinatal outcomes, timing of birth must be individualised, balancing the risk of stillbirth of the smaller twin with the benefits of prolonging the gestation for the larger twin.

2.2.5 PTB

Preterm birth (delivery <37 weeks) remains the most significant fetal complication of multiple pregnancy in terms of perinatal morbidity, mortality and cost [97]. Preterm prelabour rupture of membranes (PPROM) confers a higher chance of perinatal mortality if preterm labour ensues, due to the impact of chorioamnionitis [98]. The 2020 Mothers and Babies: Reducing Risk through Audits and Confidential Enquiries (MBRRACE) report demonstrated that the most frequent cause of perinatal loss in DC twin pregnancies was extreme preterm labour [65]. As discussed in Section 3, the etiology of spontaneous preterm labour and birth in multiple pregnancy is likely to be different to singleton pregnancy and is multifactorial, relatively poorly understood and an important field for research [99]. In a prospective study of 1,000 twin pregnancies (800 DC and 200 MC), 29% of the DC pregnancies developed a maternal or fetal condition, leading to birth before 36 weeks, whereas 34% of the MC twins were born before 34 weeks [100]. In a 2021 systematic review of 29,864 twin pregnancies, monochorionicity was found to be associated with an increased risk of preterm labour and thus PTB at <34 weeks, even if TTTS had been excluded [101].

2.2.6 Cord Prolapse

Cord prolapse is an obstetric emergency with a reported incidence varying between 0.1 and 0.6% pregnancies [60]. Multiple birth is an independent risk factor for cord prolapse, which in part relates to a lower gestational age at birth, frequent malpresentation and polyhydramnios, all of which are more common in multiple pregnancy. A 2021 study demonstrated that the rate of umbilical cord prolapse for the second twin was 1.8%. An abnormal cord insertion (marginal or velamentous) of the second twin was a significant risk factor for umbilical cord prolapse in the second stage of labour (OR: 5.05, 95% CI: 1.139–22.472, p = 0.033) [61].

2.2.7 Twin Entrapment

Twin entrapment is a rare, but serious occurrence, reported to present in approximately 1 in 1,000 twin births [62]. It occurs when fetus A is presenting breech and fetus B is cephalic, leading to interlocking of the fetal heads, and is strongly associated with hypoxia and fetal death [102]. It is more common in MA twins and nulliparous women. It is hypothesised that risks are less within parous women due to a reduction in uterine tonicity, which allows fetuses to move more freely and reduce risks of entrapment.

2.2.8 Cerebral Palsy

Both asphyxia and cerebral palsy are more common in twins than in singleton births. A 2021 multicontinental study also demonstrated the prevalence of cerebral palsy increases with plurality (twins: 6.5 per 1,000 live births (95% CI: 6.1–6.9), triplets: 17.1 (95% CI: 13.6–21.2), quadruplets: 50.7 (95% CI: 25.6–88.9)), this is mainly related to PTB [64].

2.2.9 Perinatal Mortality

The rate of neonatal mortality and stillbirth for multiple pregnancies within the UK has increased slightly over the last decade. The 2022 MBRRACE report (covering births in 2020) demonstrated an overall increase in the stillbirth and neonatal mortality rate for twins over the period 2016–20; for stillbirths, 6.16 per 1,000 total births in 2016 to 7.33 per 1,000 in 2020; and for neonatal mortality, from 5.34 to 6.18 per 1,000 livebirths [65]. Rates have been relatively static since 2020 and remain significantly higher than the rates of neonatal mortality and stillbirth in singletons [103]. There are differences in the causes of stillbirths in twins when compared to singleton births. In twins, the commonest category for the primary cause of the stillbirth is 'stillbirth with no antecedent or associated obstetric factors', followed by 'specific complications of multifetal pregnancy' or 'major congenital anomaly'. The 2021 MBRRACE report on a study of 50 twin pregnancies from 2017 found that in about 50% of baby deaths, obstetric care was poor, and that improvements in care might have reduced adverse perinatal and fetal outcomes [104].

It is known that perinatal mortality is higher in MC pregnancies than DC pregnancies with a 2.5 RR [105]. A significant proportion of this increased risk will be due to the shared placental circulation and specific fetal risks of MC twins, as described in Section 2.3. Even in the absence of these specific MC complications, studies demonstrate an increased risk in uncomplicated MC pregnancies compared to DC. A 2013 systematic review and meta-analysis demonstrated an OR for stillbirth for uncomplicated MCDA pregnancies versus DCDA of 4.2 at 32 weeks, 3.7 at 34 weeks and 8.5 at 36 weeks' gestation [106]. Data from the Southwest Thames Obstetric Research Collaborative (STORK) cohort found that while overall and early mortality was higher in MC than DC twins, there was no significant difference noted after 24 weeks' gestation. This may be due to early detection and prompt treatment of complications in MC twins, which is explored further in Section 3 [79].

A 2019 review of 25 studies reporting mortality rates in MCMA twin pregnancies demonstrated an IUD rate of 4.3% (95% CI: 2.8–6.2%) of twins at 24–30 weeks, in 1.0% (95% CI: 0.6–1.7%) at 31–2 weeks and in 2.2% (95% CI: 0.9–3.9%) at 33–4 weeks' gestation [107].

2.3 Fetal Risks Specific to MCMZ Twins

Women with MC pregnancies are also at increased risk of specific fetal complications, as shown in Table 3.

Table 3 Fetal risks specific to MC twins with associated prevalence

Fetal risks specific to MCMZ twins	Prevalence of risk within total cohort of MC twins
Conjoined twins (Section 2.3.1)	0.002%* [108]
MA twins (Section 2.3.2)	5% [109]
Selective FGR (Section 2.3.3)	10–46% [110]
TRAP sequence (Section 2.3.4)	~1% [111]
TTTS (Section 2.3.5)	10–15% [112]
Twin anemia–polycythemia sequence (TAPS) (Section 2.3.6)	5% [113]

*Total prevalence within entire pregnancy cohort (gestations)

2.3.1 Conjoined Twins

Conjoined twins represent a rare form of MA twinning, estimated to occur in around 1 in 50,000 births but approximately 1 in 200,000 live births due to a stillbirth rate of 60% [108,114]. Diagnosis is made in the first trimester by the close and fixed apposition of the fetal bodies with fusion of skin lines. Classification is guided by the most prominent fusion site, with the thoraces being the most identified (~70%) [115]. Importantly, other congenital anomalies not directly related to conjoined components are also often present (~63%) [108].

The prognosis is poor, and most conjoined twins die in utero. A review found that about 80% of cases ended in termination of pregnancy (TOP), 10.7% died in utero and only 8% continued to term. The overall outcome was found to be determined primarily by the type of conjoining, the organs shared and which surgical/nonsurgical treatment options are available [116]. Conjoined twins not requiring imminent separation surgery following delivery have a relatively good prognosis (~80% survival), compared to twins requiring immediate separation surgery postpartum (~30% survival) [115]. The determination of when to separate conjoined twins depends on how extensively the vital organs are shared between each fetus [115]. Separation of twins if there is extensive sharing of vital organs can risk death of either one or both twins. The decision on separation requires multiple clinical reviews and interprofessional effort, however, the overall decision will lie with the parents.

2.3.2 MA Twins

Monoamniotic twins are rare, with an estimated prevalence of 8 in 100,000 pregnancies (1 in 20 MC gestations) [109]. Monoamnionicity is caused by late splitting of the inner cell mass at day 9–12 so that the twins share a placenta and amniotic sac [117]. Consequently, there are usually large anastomoses connecting the fetal circulations, with close umbilical cord insertions, leading to the risk of cord entanglement.

Monoamniotic twins are at increased risk of congenital malformations, and discordant anomalies affect 15–35% of pregnancies (due to late embryonic cleavage and hemodynamic imbalances), with an increased propensity for anomalies of cardiac origin (30%) [68,117]. Monoamniotic twins are also at increased risk of IUD, as previously discussed. Mechanisms for twin demise include acute hemodynamic imbalances across the large anastomoses, severe prematurity secondary to early preterm labour and congenital abnormalities. Previously, cord entanglement was thought to play a significant role, but data suggest that although this is almost invariably present at birth in MA twins, it is only implicated in causing fetal death before 24 weeks, with other causes of death thought to be more relevant [117,118].

2.3.3 sFGR

The underlying etiology of sFGR is different to that of growth restriction in singletons and relates to unequal placental sharing. There is a wide variation in the reported incidence of sFGR within MC pregnancies, ranging between 10 and 46%, which likely relates to the historic lack of consensus on diagnostic criteria for sFGR [110].

There have been various accepted definitions for sFGR. It is defined by ISUOG as a growth discordance of 25% between twins with an EFW <10th centile in the smaller fetus [92]. The additional inclusion of a discordance in abdominal circumference (AC) >10% between twins has also been noted previously [119]. More recently, a Delphi consensus report based upon 60 expert opinions advised that for MC pregnancies, at least two out of four contributory parameters (EFW of one twin <10th centile, AC of one twin <10th centile, EFW discordance of ≥25% and umbilical artery (UA) pulsatility index (PI) of the smaller twin >95th centile) are required to diagnose sFGR [89]. However, a 2022 retrospective study on 291 MC pregnancies identified that employing this new consensus criteria increased the diagnostic rate sFGR by more than 50% compared to the ISUOG criteria, but without improving the perinatal outcomes [120]. Larger studies are required looking at these and other potential parameters to determine how best to predict prognosis in these pregnancies.

In singletons or DC pregnancies, UA Doppler waveforms are used as a marker of placental resistance. In MC pregnancies, the type and diameter of vascular anastomoses can influence outcome. Thus, a classification system (Gratacos classification – type 1, 2 or 3) based on UA Doppler waveforms in the smaller twin is now accepted and is described further in Section 3.2.3 [121]. Almost 100% of twin fetuses with type 1 sFGR survive, compared to 60% of those with type 2. Type 3 is intermediate, with survival rates of 85%, but is also very unpredictable. Sudden demise of the smaller twin without signs of deterioration occurs in 15%, followed by demise of the larger twin in half of these cases [122].

2.3.4 TRAP Sequence

Twin reversed arterial perfusion sequence is a pathology unique to MC twins, with incidence reported as 1:35,000 pregnancies and 1:100 MC twins (~1%) [111]. With advances in US and the increase in AR, there are reports of increased incidence of up to 2.6% of MZ twins [123]. It involves the presence of an abnormal cardiac structure in one fetus (acardiac) that does not pump, and consequently the affected twin becomes hemodynamically dependent upon its structurally normal co-twin, via a superficial artery-to-artery placental anastomosis (Figure 2). Thus, blood flows via the UA of the healthy 'pump' twin in a reversed direction into the UA of the co-twin via the arterio-arterial (AA) anastomosis and returns via a veno-venous (VV) anastomosis back to the pump twin. The acardiac twin's blood is thus deoxygenated, which results in abnormal development of the head and upper limbs. This oxygen-depleted blood also returns to the pump twin and can thus cause some degree of hypoxemia. Twin reversed arterial perfusion is associated with a high risk of perinatal death for the pump twin, caused by a combination of high-output cardiac failure and polyhydramnios-related PTB [111]. There is also a concern about long-term neurological sequelae for the pump twin due to chronic hypoxemia, cardiac failure and PTB.

2.3.5 TTTS

In MC pregnancies, inter-twin placental vascular anastomoses exist and enable communication between their two circulations. In 10–15% of all MC twins, a significant imbalance exists that results in the development of TTTS, usually between 16 and 26 weeks [112]. This carries particularly high perinatal morbidity and mortality rates, and accounts for approximately 20% of total stillbirths in multiple pregnancies [67].

A spectrum of TTTS exists, ranging from mild disease with isolated discordant amniotic fluid volume (AFV), to severe disease with demise of one or both twins [124]. This is explored further in Section 3.2.4. Mortality primarily relates to extreme prematurity and very LBW [125]. Prospectively, there is a three-fold

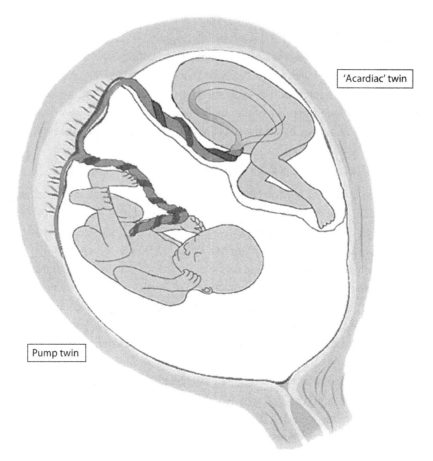

'Acardiac' twin

Pump twin

Figure 2 TRAP sequence. After Sebire N. In Ward, RH, Whittle, MJ (eds).
Multiple Pregnancy. London: RCOG Press, 1995

increased risk of congenital heart disease, as well as an increased incidence of
cerebral lesions with long-term neurological sequelae, renal morbidity and haematological disorders. Additional complications include in utero amniotic band
syndrome and in utero acquired limb ischemia [126].

2.3.6 TAPS

Twin anemia–polycythemia sequence is another disorder also restricted to MC
pregnancies, complicating 1 in 20 MCDA pregnancies. It can be spontaneous or
occur following fetoscopic laser ablation (FLA) treatment for TTTS. However,
in the absence of prenatal screening for the condition, the prevalence is suspected to be much greater [113,127]. In rare cases, TAPS has been noted to
develop following spontaneous placenta thrombosis leading to rapid succession

of fetal hydrops [128]. Complications of TAPS include severe anemia leading to hydrops in the donor, and severe polycythemia in the recipient may lead to cardiac failure and cerebral vascular accidents. Both twins are at risk of later IUD [129].

3 Management Options

3.1 Pre-pregnancy

3.1.1 AR

Over the past three decades there has been a remarkable improvement in AR, characterised by the increase in the live birth rate per transfer. However, improved pregnancy rates have been linked with concerns about increasing multiple pregnancies and the associated maternal morbidity and perinatal morbidity and mortality because of AR [130]. Consequently, international regulatory policies now recommend an elective SET (eSET) policy in almost all cases to reduce the rate of multiple birth [8,131]. This has resulted in a significant reduction in the number of two or more embryo transfer cycles performed, particularly in younger women and a reduction in the multiple birth rate in the UK following AR, as previously discussed [1,9]. However, international data show that high twin and higher-order multiple pregnancy rates still exist [4,5]. Even in developed countries, these problems persist, depending on clinical practice, funding of health services and patient demands. For example, recent data from the first registry report from China for 2016 showed a twin rate with IVF and intracytoplasmic sperm injection (ICSI) of 27.9 and 27.2%, respectively [132]. The highest twin rate from fresh IVF and ICSI was Taiwan at 35.4% and the lowest Japan at 4.2% [133].

A 2020 Cochrane review of 17 randomised controlled trials (RCT) comparing the clinical effectiveness of eSET versus DET suggests that the overall live birth rate is reduced following SET (RR: 0.67, 95% CI: 0.59–0.75). However, the cumulative live birth rate following repeated SET (two cycles of fresh SET or one cycle of fresh SET followed by one cycle of frozen SET) may be little or no different compared to a single cycle of DET (RR: 0.95, 95% CI: 0.82–1.10). The multiple pregnancy rate with repeated SET is reduced compared to a single cycle of DET (OR: 0.13, 95% CI: 0.08–0.21) (i.e., a 13% risk of multiple pregnancy with DET versus a 0–3% risk with SET) [134]. Elective SET is associated with a reduced risk of adverse outcomes such as antepartum haemorrhage (OR: 0.35, 95% CI: 0.15–0.82), LBW (OR: 0.20, 95% CI: 0.16–0.25), PTB rate (OR: 0.25, 95% CI: 0.16–0.25) and neonatal intensive care unit (NICU) admission (OR: 0.30, 95% CI: 0.14–0.66) [135]. However, only some of the excess morbidity in multiple pregnancy resulting from AR can be attributed to multiple pregnancy, as singleton pregnancies arising from AR are also associated with worse perinatal outcomes when compared to natural conception, including placental complications, hypertensive disorders and pre-natal hospitalisations [136].

More recently, a shift in practice towards delayed embryo transfer on day 5–6 (blastocyst stage), as opposed to day 2–3 (cleavage stage), has occurred in order to increase reproductive success and reduce miscarriage risk. The 2022 Cochrane review of 32 RCTs identified uncertain evidence as to whether blastocyst-stage transfer increases multiple pregnancy, while the live birth rate was significantly higher in the delayed blastocyst culture group (OR: 1.27, 95% CI: 1.06–1.51) [137]. A 2019 systematic review and meta-analysis assessed whether blastocyst transfer compared to cleavage-style transfer increased the risk of MZ or MC twinning and reported a significantly increased risk of MZ (OR: 2.16, 95% CI: 1.74–2.68) and MC (OR: 1.29, 95% CI: 1.03–1.62) pregnancies following blastocyst transfer. Conventional IVF was also associated with a statistically significantly increased risk of MZ twin pregnancy compared with ICSI (OR: 1.19, 95% CI: 1.04–1.35) and assisted hatching (OR: 1.17, 95% CI: 1.09–1.27) [138].

Counselling and Support

Thus, for couples receiving AR therapy that could result in a multiple preg-nancy, pre-pregnancy counselling and support regarding this risk is required. Both the psychological and financial effects of multiple pregnancy on a family are significant. Women should be aware of this and understand that additional support may be of value. This is a particular concern when infants are preterm with long-term neurodevelopmental complications.

SUMMARY OF MANAGEMENT OPTIONS

Pre-pregnancy

For women undergoing assisted conception:
- counsel about the risks of multiple pregnancy
- SET is recommended
- blastocyst-stage transfer results in more MZ and MC twins than cleav-age-stage transfer
- conventional IVF results in more MZ twins than ICSI or assisted hatching

3.2 Prenatal

3.2.1 General Management Options for all Twin Pregnancies

Multiple pregnancies require specialised and individualised care, and there is a consensus that this should be in specialist multidisciplinary clinics/services, with non-randomised data suggesting an improvement in perinatal outcome with this model. These clinics/services should comprise an experienced midwife and obstetrician, allowing discussion and decision-making, and access to immediate diagnostic US and multidisciplinary opinions (i.e., anaesthetic, neonatal paediatric and psychological services). This model affords timely diagnosis of any complications of multiple pregnancy along with an individualised plan of care for the prenatal, intrapartum and postnatal periods [139,140,141]. Standardised antenatal care for multiple pregnancies has been clearly shown to significantly improve maternal-fetal outcomes [142,143].

Women with multiple pregnancies require frequent antenatal visits. Not only does this facilitate early detection of potential complications but it also provides the opportunity to provide specialised prenatal counselling and support. Education and readily accessible multidisciplinary support are particularly important in this context. Parents will require specific information to help prepare for birth and postnatal care.

Parents should be encouraged to attend specific multiple-birth support group meetings, and to liaise with families who have experienced multiple birth. Useful websites, both UK and non-UK, include:

- Twins Trust: www.twinstrust.org.uk
- Multiple Births Foundation: www.multiplebirths.org.uk
- Multiples of America: https://multiplesofamerica.org/
- International Council of Multiple Birth Organisations: https://icombo.org/
- Australian Multiple Birth Association: www.amba.org.au/
- Multiples New Zealand: https://multiples.org.nz/
- Multiple Births Canada: www.multiplebirths.ca/

The following groups with multiple pregnancy are higher risk and should be managed in a tertiary care centre [54,144]:

- MCMA twin and triplet pregnancies
- MCDA and DCDA triplet pregnancies
- conjoined twins or triplets
- all higher-order pregnancies

- pregnancies complicated by any of the following:
  - discordant fetal growth
  - fetal anomaly
  - discordant fetal death
  - sFGR
  - TRAP
  - TTTS
  - TAPS

Summary of Management Options

Prenatal: Management Options for all Twin Pregnancies
General

- Specialised multidisciplinary twin/multiple pregnancy clinics/services and a standardised approach to care improve maternal and fetal outcomes.
- A tertiary centre care is recommended for:
  - MCMA twin and triplet pregnancies
  - MCDA and DCDA triplet pregnancies
  - all higher-order pregnancies
  - pregnancies complicated by discordant fetal growth, fetal anomaly, discordant fetal death, TTTS, TAPS, TRAP or sFGR
  - conjoined twins or triplets.

3.2.2 Screening and Prevention for Maternal Complications

Specific recommendations related to general antenatal care for women with multiple pregnancy relate to nutrition, anemia and risk of PTB.

Nutrition

The metabolic rate of the mother is 10% greater in multiple pregnancy, reflecting the increased nutrient demands and placental size in this setting. Evidence regarding the potential benefits of special high-calorie diets and/or specific dietary advice upon multiple pregnancy outcomes is not currently sufficient as a basis for robust recommendations [144]. Women with multiple pregnancies should therefore receive prenatal counselling regarding nutritional intake as in routine antenatal care [54], with access to a specialist dietitian if required [144].

Anemia

In view of the higher incidence of anemia and haemorrhage in women with multiple pregnancies, a full blood count should be performed at 20–4 weeks to identify whether earlier supplementation with iron or folic acid is required, in addition to that performed routinely at 28 weeks [54]. Anemia should be corrected antenatally to reduce the subsequent risk of a blood transfusion.

Hypertensive Disorders of Pregnancy

Since multifetal pregnancy is a moderate risk factor for pre-eclampsia, women with multiple pregnancy need only one additional risk factor from the following list to be recommended to take 75–150 mg/day of aspirin from 12 weeks until birth [54]:

- first pregnancy
- age 40 years or older
- pregnancy interval of more than 10 years
- body mass index (BMI) of 35 kg/m^2 or more at first visit
- family history of pre-eclampsia.

Women with major risk factors such as prior hypertension, renal impairment, diabetes or autoimmune disease would be recommended aspirin irrespective of multiple pregnancy. All women should have their blood pressure measured and urine tested for proteinuria to screen for hypertensive disorders at each antenatal appointment in twin and triplet pregnancies as per routine antenatal care [54,145].

PTB

Preterm birth is the leading cause of neonatal mortality and morbidity, and the risk of PTB is as much as 10-times higher in twins than in singletons [1]. In the 2020 MBRRACE report, PTB was the leading cause of perinatal loss in DC twins [65]. The causes of PTB for both singletons and multiples are multifactorial (Figure 3) but a significant proportion in multiples are medically indicated due to maternal and or neonatal risks (i.e., iatrogenic) [146]. The pathological causes of spontaneous PTB are similar to singletons (i.e., infection, cervical insufficiency, placental dysfunction and stress) but again may occur in greater proportions [147]. Preterm prelabour rupture of membranes complicates 7–8% of twin pregnancies at a mean gestation of 30–2 weeks (compared with 2–4% of singletons). Additionally, the uterus may have a restricted capacity to distend and permit adequate fetal growth within a multiple pregnancy, thus creating a risk for preterm labour [5]. In a prospective study of 1,000 twin pregnancies (800 DC and 200 MC), 29% of the DC pregnancies developed a maternal or fetal condition, leading to birth before 36 weeks, whereas 34% of the MC twins were born before 34 weeks [100]. In a systematic review of 29,864 twin pregnancies, monochorionicity was found to be associated with an increased

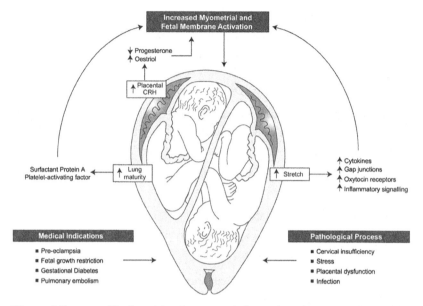

Figure 3 Factors affecting risk of preterm delivery in twins. Reproduced with permission from Stock, S, Norman, J. Preterm and term labour in multiple pregnancies. Semin Fetal Neonatal Med. 2010; 15: 336–41

risk of preterm labour and thus PTB at <34 weeks, even if TTTS had been excluded [101]. It is thus recommended that women with a multiple pregnancy are informed of the risks and symptoms and signs of PTB [54].

Predicting the Risk of Preterm Labour

Tools to assist obstetricians in predicting and stratifying the risk of preterm delivery in women with multiple pregnancy have gained increasing attention. Fetal fibronectin (fFN) measurements may be of clinical value in threatened preterm labour (i.e., symptomatic women). The National Institute for Health and Care Excellence (NICE) guidance for preterm labour and birth recommends in symptomatic women considering fFN testing to determine the likelihood of birth within 48 hours for women who are 30^{+0} weeks pregnant or more, if cervical length (CL) measurement is indicated, but is not available or not acceptable [148]. For asymptomatic presentations, the accuracy of fFN testing in multiple gestations is inconclusive, as reported in a 2018 meta-analysis by dos Santos et al. [149]. However, the studies in this review used qualitative fFN. Since the systematic review, a study by Shennan et al. demonstrated that quantitative fFN (qfFN) can be used to predict PTB <30 weeks' gestation in asymptomatic women and that CL strengthens the prediction. This data have been incorporated into the QUIPP app, which combines qfFN, CL and woman's risk factors, and evaluated in a cohort including twins

[150,151]. At present, NICE guidance does not recommend the use of fFN alone in screening asymptomatic women with multiple pregnancy [54,152]. In September 2024 the manufacture ceased production of fetal fibronectin for the UK market and thus it will no longer be available.

Cervial length is not routinely measured in women with multiple pregnancies in order to screen for risk of PTB in an asymptomatic population. A 2016 meta-analysis of 4,409 asymptomatic twin pregnancies demonstrated a significant and non-linear relationship between the gestational age at screening and CL measurement on the gestational age at birth [153]. Earlier screening ($\leq 18^{+0}$ weeks) was most predictive of PTB prior to 28 weeks, whereas later screening ($>22^{+0}$ weeks) was more predictive of delivery at 28^{+1}–36^{+0} weeks' gestation [153]. Serial CL measurements provide some promise for predicting the risk of PTB. However, a distinction between screening all multiple gestation pregnancies (a large cost implication) or only subgroups of patients with certain predisposing risk factors needs to be established to not over-investigate and over-intervene. The current recommendation of NICE is that CL measurement should not routinely be used as a screening method [54]. In 2024 NICE updated their guidance to recommend that women with a twin or triplet pregnancy are offered a single cervical length scan between 16 and 20 weeks [54].

Prevention of Preterm Labour

In the NICE Twin and Triplet Pregnancy guideline, based on available evidence, the following interventions are not routinely advised in the context of PTB prevention in multiple pregnancy [54]:

- bed rest at home or in hospital
- intramuscular (IM) progesterone
- Arabin pessary
- cervical cerclage
  - history indicated
  - ultrasound indicated
  - physically indicated
- oral tocolytics.

The Society for Maternal–Fetal Medicine (SMFM) and ACOG also do not recommended restriction of activity, use of tocolytics or cervical cerclage for prevention of PTB (history and US indicated) based solely on the indication of multiple gestation, however, physically indicated cerclage should be considered on a case-by-case basis [154,155].

Bed-rest

Historically, bed-rest has been seen as a useful approach to reduce the risk of PTB. However, a recent Cochrane review of six RCTs evaluating the role of complete or partial bed-rest to reduce the incidence of PTB in twin and triplet pregnancy found no evidence to support its use [156]. Prolonged bed-rest is also associated with an increased risk of venous thromboembolism and worsening maternal mental illness [73].

Progestogens

There has been much research interest in vaginal progesterone for the prevention of PTB in twin pregnancy. There have been several systematic reviews and individual patient data (IPD) assessing the evidence and different subgroups of women that have informed current guidelines. A 2019 Cochrane systematic analysis, which included 17 studies (4,773 women), concluded that overall, for women with a multiple pregnancy, the administration of progesterone (either IM or vaginal) does not appear to be associated with a reduction in risk of PTB (<34 weeks) or improved neonatal outcomes [157]. A 2017 updated IPD meta-analysis assessed individual patient data outcomes for 303 asymptomatic women with a twin gestation and sonographic short cervix (≤25 mm) in the mid-trimester (159 assigned to vaginal progesterone and 144 assigned to placebo/no treatment) and their 606 fetuses/infants from six RCTs [158]. The authors concluded that vaginal progesterone treatment, compared with placebo, is associated with a statistically significant reduction in the risk of PTB <33 weeks (31.4 vs 43.1%, RR: 0.69, 95% CI: 0.51–0.93, moderate-quality evidence). Moreover, vaginal progesterone administration was found to be associated with a significant decrease in the risk of PTB <35, <34, <32 and <30 weeks (RRs range: 0.47–0.83), NND (RR: 0.53, 95% CI: 0.35–0.81), RDS (RR: 0.70, 95% CI: 0.56–0.89), composite neonatal morbidity and mortality (RR: 0.61, 95% CI: 0.34–0.98), use of mechanical ventilation (RR: 0.54, 95% CI: 0.36 –0.81) and BW <1,500 g (RR: 0.53, 95% CI: 0.35–0.80) (all moderate-quality evidence). Some of the significant findings reported in this analysis (PTB <33 weeks, NND) became statistically non-significant when the sensitivity analysis was restricted to trials with adequate blinding of patients, clinical staff and outcome assessors. However, the sensitivity analyses did not substantially change the magnitude and direction of effect sizes obtained in the overall analysis. It should be noted that 74% of the sample size included within this review was provided by a single study that has now been retracted online [159].

Thus ACOG, SMFM and Royal Australian and New Zealand College of Obstetricians and Gynaecologists (RANZCOG) currently do not recommend the use of vaginal progesterone for preventing PTB in twin pregnancies [155,160,161].

In 2024 NICE considered the evidence for progesterone and updated their guidance to include advice for management of women identified with a short cervix on ultrasound. This included offering progesterone 200mg vaginal capsules once a day when the cervical length was 25 mm or less, until 34 weeks [54]. The Evaluating Progestogens for Preventing Preterm Birth International Collaborative (EPPPIC) meta-analysis published in 2021 compared vaginal, IM or oral progesterone with a control or with each other in asymptomatic women at risk of PTB [162]. Eight trials on multiple gestations were included, mostly including women without additional risk factors. Within the study vaginal progesterone did not reduce PTB before 34 weeks (eight trials, 2,046 women, RR: 1.01, 95% CI: 0.84–1.20) nor did IM progesterone for twins or triplets (eight trials, 2,253 women: 1.04, 0.92–1.18) [162]. Moreover, PPROM was increased with IM progesterone exposure in multiple gestations (rupture <34 weeks, RR: 1.59, 95% CI: 1.15–2.22) [162]. However, the authors found no consistent evidence of benefit or harm for other outcomes with either vaginal or IM progesterone. A 2021 study by Rehal et al., which was not included within the EPPPIC study, examined 1,194 twin pregnancies randomised to either vaginal progesterone or placebo [163]. Findings were similar with EPPPIC in that there was no overall reduction in PTB with the administration of vaginal progesterone. However, a 2021 post hoc time-to-event analysis suggested that vaginal progesterone may reduce the risk of spontaneous PTB <32 weeks in twin pregnancies with a CL <30mm, although it may increase the risk of PTB if CL ≥30mm [163].

In a 2022 updated meta-analysis of six placebo-controlled studies, the use of vaginal progesterone for asymptomatic twin gestations with a short cervix (≤25 mm) detected sonographically demonstrated a statistically significant reduction in PTB <33 weeks (38.5 vs 55.8%, RR: 0.60, 95% CI: 0.38–0.95, p = 0.03, I^2 = 14%) [164]. Significant reductions in PTB were also seen at <34, <32, <30 and <28 weeks in groups administered with vaginal progesterone. However significant reductions in PTB were not seen for <35, <36 and <37 weeks' gestation. A declining trend was also seen in composite neonatal morbidity and mortality [164]. The PROSPECT study is an eagerly awaited RCT that has been ongoing since November 2015, looking at the use of vaginal progesterone (200 mg/day) or cervical pessary compared a placebo to reduce the rate of PTB in twin gestations with a CL <30 mm between gestation weeks 16 and 23 [165]. The current recruitment target for this study is 630 participants. The ISUOG guideline for the role of US in the prediction of spontaneous PTB was updated in 2022 and concluded that the prophylactic use of progesterone is not recommended in unselected pregnancies but that it could be considered in twin pregnancy with CL ≤25 mm [166].

There is limited available evidence of the potential benefit of IM progesterone for twin pregnancies with a short cervix. A 2016 Cochrane review revealed that the risk of PTB <34 weeks' gestation was greater in the IM progesterone group compared to placebo (RR: 1.54, 95% CI: 1.06–2.26, 399 pregnancies, two studies; low-quality evidence) [157]. Given the insufficient evidence for IM progesterone, it is currently not recommended for use in PTB prevention.

Arabin Pessary

The value of Arabin cervical pessaries for PTB prevention in multiple pregnancy is also uncertain. In singleton pregnancies, there is evidence to suggest a potential benefit in relation to timing of delivery, and that treatment is overall well tolerated [167]. Whether this therapy significantly reduces neonatal morbidity and mortality, however, is less clear. Specifically, within the context of multiple pregnancy, the ProTwin multicentre RCT in the Netherlands published in 2013 measured the effect of cervical pessaries directly upon neonatal outcome [168]. Of 808 women included in the analysis (401 pessary group, 407 control group), 53 (13%) in the pessary group had a poor perinatal outcome, compared with 55 (14%) in the control group (RR: 0.98, 95% CI: 0.69–1.39). Prophylactic use of a cervical pessary in all-risk multiple pregnancies was not found to reduce poor perinatal outcome (stillbirth, periventricular leukomalacia, severe RDS, bronchopulmonary dysplasia, intraventricular haemorrhage, necrotising enterocolitis, proven sepsis and NND). Planned subgroup analysis in women with a CL <25th centile (<38 mm) (n = 78 pessary group, 55 control group) did find that the pessary significantly reduced the frequency of poor perinatal outcome and very preterm delivery [168]. The results from the ProTwin trial have been corroborated by the 2016 PECEP-Twins trial, whereby a cervical pessary placement for a CL ≤25 mm demonstrated a significant reduction in rate of spontaneous PTB prior to 34 weeks compared to expectant management (11/68 (16.2%) vs 26/66 (39.4%), RR: 0.41, 95% CI: 0.22–0.76) [169].

Data from a 2016 open-label international RCT evaluating prophylactic cervical Arabin pessary insertion from 20 to 24^{+6} weeks' gestation until elective removal or delivery versus expectant management in twin pregnancies (n = 1180 women) found no difference in spontaneous early PTB at <34 weeks (RR: 1.054, 95% CI: 0.787–1.413, p = 0.722), perinatal death (RR: 0.908, 95% CI: 0.553–1.491, p = 0.702), adverse neonatal outcome (RR: 1.094, 95% CI: 0.851–1.407, p = 0.524) or neonatal therapy (RR: 1.040, 95% CI: 0.871–1.242, p = 0.701) [170]. Comparing this to the ProTwin trail there were different cut-offs used for reduced CL (22 and 38 mm, respectively) which may explain the different conclusions.

This was similarly the case for a 2018 open RCT of 357 pregnant women (24^{+0}–33^{+6} weeks) who had not delivered 48 hours after a threatened preterm labour episode and had a short cervix remaining (≤25 mm at 24^{+0}–29^{+6} weeks; ≤15 mm at 30^{+0}–33^{+6} weeks). No significant differences between the pessary and routine management groups were observed in the spontaneous PTB rate <34 weeks (19/177 (10.7%) in the pessary group vs 24/175 (13.7%) in the control group; RR 0.78; 95% CI, 0.45–1.38) [171]. A systematic review that assessed the effectiveness of cervical pessary in the prevention of PTB in multiple pregnancies with a short cervix (<25 mm) found no benefit of using cervical pessary in the prevention of PTB, BW <1,500 g, <2,500 g, adverse neonatal events and fetal/NND in twin pregnancies with a short cervix. The authors concluded that more RCTs are required in this area [172].

In response to this call, the STOPPIT-2 RCT was completed in 2021. This was a multicentre open-label RCT and screened 2,228 twin pregnancies for a short CL between weeks 18^{+0} and 20^{+6}. Women with a CL ≤35mm were assigned to either an insertion of pessary and standard care, or standard care alone. The Arabin pessary was associated with 18.4% rate of PTB <34 weeks compared with 20.6% following standard care alone (AOR: 0.87, 95% CI: 0.55–1.38, p = 0.54) [173]. The evidence remains that the use of the Arabin pessary for PTB prevention has limited efficacy.

Cervical Cerclage

Cervical cerclage for any indication (history, US or physical exam) is not routinely recommended since the effectiveness and safety of this procedure in multiple gestations remains controversial. This recommendation is mainly based on a 2014 Cochrane review (five trials of average to above average quality, n = 128 multiple pregnancies, 122 twins and six triplets) that investigated whether cervical cerclage improved perinatal outcomes (perinatal death and/or serious neonatal morbidity) specifically in multiple gestations identified as high risk of pregnancy loss according to maternal history alone, US findings of 'short cervix' or physical exam changes in the cervix. No statistically significant differences in perinatal deaths (19.2 vs 9.5%, RR: 1.74, 95% CI: 0.92–3.28) or serious neonatal morbidity (15.8 vs 13.6%, RR: 0.96, 95% CI: 0.13–7.10) were identified, but this in part reflects the low participant numbers included [174].

History-indicated cerclages can be placed for patients who have predisposing risk factors that may increase the propensity of these patients to develop future cervical insufficiency and subsequently deliver preterm. A retrospective cohort study in 2019 of 82 twin pregnancies with a prior history of PTB at 20–36 weeks' gestation were split to either having a history-indicated cerclage or expectant management. The rates of spontaneous PTB <24 weeks (2.4 vs 19.5%, OR: 0.10, 95% CI: 0.01–0.87, p = 0.03), <28 weeks (12.2 vs 34.1%, OR: 0.27, 95% CI: 0.09–0.84, p = 0.03), <32 weeks (22.0 vs 56.1%, OR: 0.22, 95% CI: 0.08–0.58, p = 0.003) and <34 weeks (34.1 vs 82.9%, OR: 0.11, 95% CI: 0.04–0.30, p <0.0001) were significantly lower in the cerclage group than in the control group [175]. This study demonstrated the potential positive implications that history-indicated cerclage can have in twin gestations on reducing the rate of PTB.

The detection of a short cervix on US, in the absence of symptomatology suggesting threatened preterm labour may warrant the placement of a cervical cerclage. A 2019 meta-analysis of 16 studies reporting on the placement of a cervical cerclage following incidental finding of a CL <15 mm on US in twin pregnancies demonstrated a significant prolongation of pregnancy (mean difference of 3.89 weeks' gestation, 95% CI: 2.19–5.59, p = 0.000, I^2 = 0%) and a reduction of PTB <34 weeks' gestation (RR: 0.57, 95% CI: 0.43–0.75, p = 0.000, I^2 = 0%) and <32 weeks' gestation (RR: 0.61, 95% CI: 0.41–0.90, p = 0.010, I^2 = 0%), compared to those pregnancies expectantly managed [176]. There was, however, some criticism of this study, as much of the data were derived from retrospective cohort studies rather than high-quality RCTs. There are two RCTs that are in the recruitment phase that will examine the potential benefit of cervical cerclage for twin pregnancies with a short cervix [177,178]. These may provide valuable recommendations towards the potential clinical efficacy of this intervention, but until then, based on the current evidence, a US-indicated cervical cerclage is not routinely recommended.

Cervical cerclages can also be placed in situations whereby physical examination indicates evidence of a dilated cervix, in the absence of symptoms of preterm labour. Li et al. demonstrated a significant prolongation of pregnancy (mean difference of 6.78 weeks, 95% CI: 5.32–8.24; p <0.0001), significant reduction of PTB <34, <32, <28 and <24 weeks' gestation by 40–65%, and significant improvement in the perinatal outcomes for twin pregnancies presenting with a dilated cervix >10 mm between 14 and 26 weeks' gestation [176]. An RCT published in 2020 was concluded prematurely as there was a demonstrated significant benefit within the intervention arm [179]. The insertion of a physical indicated cerclage in twin gestation was associated with a reduction in PTB at less than 28 weeks of 50%, with an overall reduction in perinatal mortality by 78%. The study also demonstrated a significant reduction in PTB at all gestations when cerclage was used in a combination with tocolytics (indomethacin) and antibiotics [179]. The updated 2022 ISUOG practice guideline for US in PTB prediction recommends a consideration of physical examination cerclage in twin pregnancies with a short cervix when in combination with antibiotics and tocolytics [166].

Use of Corticosteroids

The use of corticosteroids in twin pregnancy is not routinely recommended, unless targeted in the context of threatened PTB, PPROM or intended iatrogenic early PTB [54]. Whether corticosteroids are as effective in preventing RDS as in singleton pregnancies is uncertain. The benefits and harms of antenatal cortico-steroids at later preterm gestations are an important area of research.

Management of Threatened Preterm Labour

Of those women who present with symptoms suggestive of preterm labour, only 22–9% subsequently deliver within seven days [152,180]. In the setting of PTB, the timely administration of antenatal steroids is crucial. The 2018 EPIPIAGE-2 study demonstrated a significant reduction in perinatal mortal-ity, periventricular leukomalacia and intraventricular haemorrhage in twin neonates that were delivered within seven days of the completed course of steroid regime [181]. However, as it is difficult to predict PTB, it is important to educate women about the signs and symptoms of preterm labour so that they can present early, and corticosteroids can be given in time to optimise efficacy.

Infection/inflammation is commonly associated with PTB, in particular at <30 weeks' gestation. Given the association between PPROM and intrauterine infection, current guidance endorses the routine use of antibiotics for women with PPROM [182]. In singletons, this is shown to have significant short-term value in terms of reduced infection rates, improved latency to delivery and early perinatal outcome, but the long-term benefits are not proven [183]. Studies specifically evaluating prophylactic antibiotic use in twins are limited, the evidence regarding singletons guides current practice [184].

Antenatal Magnesium Sulphate

A Cochrane review involving 6,145 babies concluded that antenatal therapy administered to women at risk of PTB substantially reduced the risk of moderate to severe cerebral palsy in their offspring. Subgroup analysis comparing single-ton and twin outcomes found no significant difference. Magnesium sulphate in twins at risk of PTB is therefore recommended for neuroprotection when delivery is anticipated, and no contraindications exist. [185].

Tocolytics

The value of tocolytics is more controversial in multiple pregnancy with limited published data on their use [186]. Tocolytic therapy for 48 hours may enable corticosteroid administration. Beyond this their utility is unproven, and certainly the potential risks of therapy require consideration by an experienced obstetrician. There has been an RCT underway since 2016 comparing the use of Atosiban (oxytocin inhibitor) versus nifedipine (calcium channel blocker) for the manage-ment of preterm labour in twin pregnancies [187]. Its primary and secondary outcomes include duration of labour and infant morbidity.

Delayed Delivery of the Second Twin

After delivery of the first fetus during a very early PTB or second-trimester miscarriage, delay in delivery may be an effective management option to increase the chance of survival of the remaining fetus(es). Meta-analysis of 492 pregnancies (432 twins (88%), 56 triplets (11%), three quadruplets and one quintuplets) found that a delayed-interval delivery significantly improved the perinatal survival of remaining fetus(es) compared with the first-born (OR: 5.2, 95% CI: 2.95–9.25), before 20 weeks (OR: 6.32, 95% CI: 1.99–20.13) between 20 and 23^{+6} weeks (OR: 3.31, 95% CI: 1.95–5.63) and >24 weeks (OR: 1.92, 95% CI: 1.21–3.05), in DCDA (OR: 14.89, 95% CI: 6.19–35.8), and in unselected triplet pregnancy (OR: 2.33, 95% CI: 1.02–5.32) [188]. No significant difference in short- or long-term neonatal morbidities between the first-born and the remaining fetus(es) was identified. Serious maternal morbidity was however reported in 39% of pregnancies after delayed-interval delivery.

SUMMARY OF MANAGEMENT OPTIONS

Screening for and Prevention of Maternal Complications

Nutrition

• Routine antenatal counselling regarding nutritional intake is recommended, and women with multiple pregnancy should be made specifically aware of the increased metabolic demands associated with multiple pregnancy, though there is no evidence to support advocating an increased calorific intake.

Anemia

• Perform a full blood count at 20–4 weeks to identify whether earlier supplementation with iron or folic acid is required, in addition to that performed routinely at 28 weeks.

Hypertensive Disease

• Screen for hypertensive disease with blood pressure and urinalysis at antenatal appointments.
• Assess risk of hypertensive disorders and prescribe low-dose aspirin (75–150 mg/day) for women with two or more of the following risk factors:
  • first pregnancy

(cont.)

- age ≥40 years
- pregnancy interval >10 years
- BMI ≥35 kg/m^2 at first visit
- family history of pre-eclampsia.

Preterm Labour

- Women should receive clear, timely counselling and support regarding their significantly increased risk of PTB.

Predicting the Risk of Preterm Labour

- Fetal fibronectin: not routinely recommended in asymptomatic women with multiple pregnancy in the UK; should be reserved for use in symptomatic women.
- Women with twin or triplet pregnancy in the UK can be offered a CL measurement between 16–20 weeks.

Prevention of Preterm Labour

- There is no evidence of benefit of routine use of bed-rest or oral tocolytics.
- There is conflicting evidence of benefit of cervical cerclage (indicated by history, cervical US or vaginal examination), Arabin pessaries or IM progesterone.
- In the UK vaginal progesterone can be offered to women with a twin or triplet pregnancy and a short cervix (</= 25mm).
- Only use corticosteroids with an additional risk of preterm delivery (e.g., threatened PTL, PPROM, elective preterm delivery).

Management of Threatened Preterm Labour

- Counsel women about the higher risk of PTB, ask them to be vigilant for early symptoms of preterm labour and encourage prompt self-referral if PTL is suspected.
- Routinely use antibiotics with PPROM, although the evidence is from studies in singleton pregnancies.
- Give magnesium sulphate if preterm delivery is anticipated.
- Give corticosteroids.
- The use of tocolytics is controversial.
- More data are needed to allow recommendations about delaying the delivery of the second twin.

3.2.3 Prenatal Surveillance

Dating and Chorionicity

As soon as a multiple pregnancy is identified, the gestational age, amnionicity and chorionicity should be documented with US. This enables appropriate planning of prenatal care and surveillance as well as allowing informed counselling of the risks of the multiple pregnancy for the parents. Knowledge of chorionicity is also important in the event of the need for invasive diagnostic procedures or counselling in the event of discordance (anomaly or growth).

Assessment of size for dating purposes is performed in the first trimester at the same time as chorionicity and amnionicity assessment whenever possible, using crown rump length (CRL) as the recommended measure. This should be performed when the CRL is between 45 and 84 mm (i.e., 11^{+0}–13^{+6} weeks) [92]. Crown rump length discrepancy within the first trimester is a common finding when scanning multiple gestations [189]. To assist identification of early fetal growth pathology, the larger fetus measurements are generally used to estimate gestational age [54,92]. When twin pregnancy follows IVF, gestational age is decided by using oocyte retrieval date and adding 14 days.

Small CRL differences between twins within the first trimester may appear to be physiological, however, larger discrepancies may be of pathological origin and warrant a referral to fetal medicine specialist for a detailed assessment in view of worsening perinatal outcome [88]. This has been confirmed by a 2020 cohort study of 6,225 twin pregnancies that demonstrated an increased CRL discordance is associated with increased fetal and perinatal death [88]. Crown rump length discrepancy in the first trimester of 10 mm represents a significant growth discrepancy and is predictive of subsequent EFW discordance [73,83,190]. Management of CRL discordance is determined by chorionicity. In MC twins, invasive testing should occur when additional anomalies are co-existing, however, discordance should prompt more intense fetal surveillance due to the high risk associated with sFGR secondary to unequal placental vascular sharing (AUC: 0.89) [191]. In DC twins, a reduced fetal size may present as the first sign of a congenital anomaly, as the risk of fetal anomalies is greater in DC compared to MC twins, thus CRL discordance should prompt detail second-trimester assessment, as well as invasive testing [92,191].

The accuracy of second-trimester estimation of dating by size measurement is acceptable if required, and the best estimate is obtained by using head circumference (HC), AC and femur length in combination [83]. For women having the dating scan performed after 14 weeks, the larger HC should be used to date the pregnancy [92].

Chorionicity should be determined at the time the twin pregnancy is detected. This is best performed before 14 weeks' gestation. After this time, distinguishing US features become more difficult to identify. Accuracy rates for determining chorionicity at first-trimester US (compared to pathological examination) are up to 96% with transabdominal US and 100% with transvaginal [192,193]. Prior to 10 weeks' gestation, a single gestational sac containing two live fetuses can indicate the presence of MC twins, compared with two gestational sacs with individual live fetal poles suggesting DC twins [194]. Between 10 and 14 weeks, the number of placental masses, a lambda sign or T-sign, membrane thickness and sex discordance should be assessed to elicit chorionicity [54]. It is recommended that a US image is kept in the maternity records for future reference [92]. If only one placenta is visualised, the presence of an extension of chorionic tissue (lambda sign) suggests dichorionicity, and its absence (T-sign), monochorionicity (Figure 4) [194,195]. Additionally, a thin inter-twin membrane is associated with MC twins, whereas an echogenic and thick membrane suggests DC twins. There are several pitfalls during the dating scan that can lead to difficulty when determining chorionicity. In advancing gestation, the appearance of the lambda sign can become less prominent. A 2016 meta-analysis of more than 2,000 twins reported a diagnostic accuracy of the lambda signs of 99% prior to 14 weeks' gestation for diagnosing DC twins, whereas by 20 weeks' gestation, the accuracy fell substantially to 7% [196,197]. Furthermore, there are several anatomical variations of the membrane-placental junction (MPJ) that can mimic a lambda sign. Cord insertion at the MPJ may resemble a lambda sign, however, the use of colour flow Doppler can help to clarify diagnosis [198]. A haematoma at the MPJ can also mimic a fake twin peak sign, however, a continuous scan along the entire length of the MPJ can help differentiate whether or not there are two sacs [199]. In very rare circumstances, there can be co-existence of a T and lambda sign, representing a hybrid placentation constituting both MC and DC characteristics [194]. To date, there have only been three such cases reported.

Diagnosis of MA twins within the early first trimester can include assessing the number of yolk sacs, with approximately two-thirds having the presence of a single yolk sac, and one-third two yolk sacs, similar to DA twins [200]. Thus, the presence of an MA pregnancy has to be confirmed at the 11–14-week scan and is initially demonstrated by the lack of a dividing membrane on US and a transvaginal US may be required. The cords can also be assessed by pulsed-wave Doppler looking for the presence of cord entanglement [92,94]. Cord entanglement is detected when two distinct arterial waveform patterns with different heart rates are observed within the same sampling gate [92].

MC twins are MZ and thus concordant for fetal sex with discordant sex pregnancies being DZ. Very rarely there can be discordant sex MC pregnancies

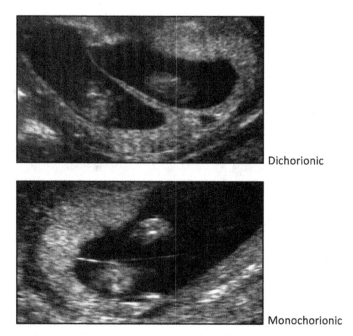

Dichorionic

Monochorionic

Figure 4 First-trimester US determination of chorionicity: DC showing lambda sign; MC showing T-sign. From Ward, RH, Whittle, MJ (eds). Multiple Pregnancy. London: RCOG Press, 1995

secondary to sex chromosome abnormalities (X/XY mosaicism, XX/XY mosaicism), genital malformations of one fetus or DZ twins forming an MC placenta [194,195]. For like-sex DC twin pregnancies, 20% will be MZ, and in these instances, zygosity can only be determined by DNA fingerprinting. It is not routine in the UK to offer this. In certain circumstances it may be required either prenatally (e.g., to determine individual genetic risk or to demonstrate dichorionicity in the presence of fetal compromise) or postnatally (e.g., to determine genetic risk, transplantation compatibility).

There has also been much recent interest in developing a systematic twin labelling system for US assessment. Determination of gestational sac position and orientation, namely, lateral (left and right) or vertical (upper and lower), is now recommended to facilitate the accuracy of serial fetal antenatal assessment and should be clearly documented in the woman's case notes [54,92]. This is considered more reliable than previous techniques that utilised fetal position relative to the maternal cervix, which is changeable and thus potentially misleading both antenatally and at the time of delivery [201]. Gestational sac position cannot be used, however, for MA pregnancies.

Twins of Unknown Chorionicity

With the advent of first-trimester scanning, the incidence of unknown chorionicity has declined rapidly. Pregnancies where this has not been accurately determined, particularly those with the same-sex and discordant growth, present a challenge. An/oligohydramnios can make the lambda sign unreliable. In this situation, 30% of twins will be MC and chorionicity should be assessed by detection of an AA anastomosis with the characteristic bidirectional waveform, DNA determination of zygosity by amniocentesis and/or identification of the cord insertion at the inter-twin membrane. Where chorionicity cannot be accurately determined, the pregnancy should be managed as an MC pregnancy [54,92].

Fetal Abnormality Screening and Diagnosis

Screening for both structural abnormalities and aneuploidy uses the same methods as for singleton pregnancies. The introduction of widespread first-trimester US and the measurement of NT has afforded women with multiple pregnancies the option of aneuploidy screening that provides a fetus-specific risk in DC pregnancies and pregnancy risk in MC pregnancies. While knowledge of chorionicity is important when considering invasive procedures and interventions, it is zygosity that determines aneuploidy risk. Before embarking on any screening or diagnostic test, parents must be adequately counselled about the possibility of a discordant anomaly and the implications of a positive result. In the case of discordant structural or chromosomal anomaly, there are essentially three management options: conservative, selective feticide (see Section 3.2.4) or termination of the whole pregnancy. Women with a triplet pregnancy should be counselled about the greater risks of aneuploidy, the increased false-positive rates for screening and thus potential need for invasive testing with greater risks for the pregnancy and the potential interventions (e.g., SR with physical risks and psychological implications) [54].

NT

At the first-trimester US scan, NT measurement for aneuploidy is offered to parents [145]. In MC twin pregnancies there is an increased risk of discordant NT measurements and an increased false-positive rate for screening. This is because discordant NT measurements may represent early manifestations of other MC pregnancy complications such as TTTS [202]. However, NT measurement is the only technique that allows an individual risk to be assigned, allowing for targeted fetal karyotyping and selection of 'low-risk' fetuses in the context of MFPR. For twins where there is a vanished twin with a remaining measurable fetal pole, triplets and higher-order multiples, the only form of first-trimester screening available is NT alone or combined with maternal age.

Discrepancy in NT in twin gestations has also been associated with adverse perinatal outcomes. A discordance of 20% between fetuses should prompt the same management options in MC and DC twins as in CRL discrepancies [191].

Combined Test

The combined screening test (NT, β-human chorionic gonadotropin (β-hCG), pregnancy-associated plasma protein A (PAPP-A)) is recommended by the NICE in twin pregnancies in the first trimester, ideally between weeks 11 and 12 [54]. Women with a multiple pregnancy should be adequately counselled regarding the greater likelihood of Trisomy 21 (Down Syndrome) before screening is performed. The potential screening options available should also be explained, and their associated sensitivities and false-positive rates. In a 2014 review of twin pregnancies undergoing the combined screening, the sensitivity and specificity for trisomy 21 were 86.2% (95% CI: 72.8–93.6) and 95.2% (95% CI: 94.2–96.0) for DC twins, while the corresponding figures for MC twins were 87.4% (95% CI: 52.6–97.7) and 95.4% (95% CI: 94.3–96.3), respectively. In comparison, sensitivity was 89% for singletons for the same 5% false-positive rate [203]. Women who have a 1:150 or greater risk should be referred to a fetal medicine specialist in a tertiary-level fetal medicine centre [54].

Second-Trimester Serum Screening

Where first-trimester screening is not able to be offered, second-trimester serum screening may be offered in the form of the quadruple test. The quadruple test can be offered between 14^{+2} and 20^{+0} weeks' gestation and measures levels of alpha-fetoprotein, human chorionic gonadotropin (hCG), unconjugated estriol and inhibin A. The screening performance for multiple pregnancy is worse when using the quadruple test, particularly with DC twins, and it is not currently recommended for screening in triplet pregnancies and higher-order multiples [54].

Non-invasive Prenatal Testing

Cell-free fetal DNA-based non-invasive prenatal testing (NIPT) has a high-test accuracy in singleton pregnancies, but a lower test accuracy in twin pregnancies. Failure rates are reported to be three-times higher in twin pregnancies than in singletons, with AR and raised maternal weight noted to be contributing factors [204]. A recent prospective multicentre study of 1,000 twins pooled its data with 11 additional studies that were previously published within the literature to identify the screening performance of using cell-free fetal DNA (cffDNA) for common trisomies (trisomy 21, 18, 13). The detection rate and false-positive rate were 95% (95% CI: 90–9) and 0.09% (95% CI: 0.03–0.19) for Trisomy 21, whilst 82% (95% CI: 66–93) and 0.08% (95% CI: 0.02–0.18) for Trisomy 18 [205]. Only five cases of

Trisomy 13 were detected, which yielded an average detection rate of 80% and false-positive rate of 0.13%; however, CIs could not be calculated due to the small sample size [205]. The worse test performance is believed to be because testing in DZ twins relies on differentiating and quantifying DNA molecules from three different sources (two non-identical twins and the mother) as opposed to just two (two identical twins or a single fetus and the mother). In DZ twins, discordance is a significant issue, as only one fetus is likely to be affected. The cffDNA fraction can vary between DZ twins nearly two-fold, which means that the cffDNA fraction from the affected fetus may be below the threshold of 4% required for testing while the unaffected twin may contribute a high cffDNA fraction; therefore, the total cffDNA fraction may appear satisfactory and produce a false-negative (low-risk) result [73,206,207].

Monozygotic twins produce identical DNA molecules and therefore should be treated as singletons during this screening test. Whilst NIPT should be easier, there is the issue of confirming chorionicity to be confident in the results. However, a small proof-of-principle study (n = 8) has demonstrated that it is possible to determine chorionicity non-invasively using cffDNA, although this needs further validation [208]. There is also the problem of single twin demise and vanishing twin, whereby the cffDNA remains within the mother's circulation. Studies predict that it remains within the maternal circulation for at least eight weeks and up to 15 weeks, and consequently has been attributed to result in 42% of the confirmed false-positive results [209,210,211].

As with all cffDNA NIPT, the ethical implications of the results also need to be considered, particularly in the case of twin discordance and potential select-ive feticide, which may not be sufficiently acknowledged by women who see NIPT as a routine blood test. Within the UK, the National Screening Committee (NSC) implemented the routine use of cffDNA as a secondary screening tool in 2020 for twin pregnancies receiving a >1 in 150 trisomy risk result from combined screening [212], in the same way it is offered as a contingent test in singleton pregnancies. The International Society of Prenatal Diagnosis (ISPD) and ACOG recommend its use in twin pregnancies [213,214].

Screening for Fetal Abnormality

If the woman consents, US should be performed between 18^{+0} and 20^{+6} weeks to detect structural anomalies. This includes extended cardiac views, namely, the four-chamber view, the left and right ventricular outflow tracts, the three-vessel view and the transverse arch view. In principle, this is no different to standard antenatal care with singleton pregnancies [145,212].

Invasive Prenatal Diagnosis

The chance of being offered invasive testing and the likelihood of complications associated with these procedures are both increased in the context of a multiple pregnancy. The complexity of counselling, performing the technique and management options necessitates that they be performed in a fetal medicine referral centre. The objectives when performing invasive testing in multiple pregnancies are:

• determination of chorionicity
• detailed US examination to determine fetal gender
• mapping/documentation of fetal position, placental site, septal site and cord insertions
• accurate and detailed labelling of samples with details of fetus and needle insertion site.

Some guidelines recommend chorionic villus sampling (CVS) as the preferred technique in DC pregnancies as it can be performed earlier and thus facilitate earlier intervention if needed [92]. In DC twins, both placentas should be sampled with a separate needle. In the case of fused placentas in DC twins or if chorionicity is doubtful, each side of the placenta should be sampled accordingly [73]. In MC twins, only one sample is usually required, notwithstanding rare cases of discordant karyotypes in MZ twins. For amniocentesis, ideally both amniotic sacs should be sampled, however, in cases where there are no detected fetal anomalies and concordant growth, a single sample from one amniotic sac may be considered.

Systematic review evidence for fetal loss following invasive testing suggests a rate of 2.0% (95% CI: 0.0–6.5%) for CVS compared with 1.8% (95% CI: 0.3–4.2%) in those not undergoing CVS. For amniocentesis, the rate was 2.4% (95% CI: 1.4–3.6%) and 2.4% (95% CI: 0.9–4.6%) for twin gestations not undergoing amniocentesis [215]. This review and a 2021 retrospective study investigating pregnancy loss after CVS demonstrate that the risk of fetal loss following amniocentesis and CVS in twins is lower than reported previously and the rate of fetal loss before 24 weeks' gestation, or within four weeks after the procedure, does not differ from the background risk in twin pregnancy not undergoing invasive prenatal testing [215,216]. There is a lack of evidence related to the risks of increasing number of needle insertions [215].

A high level of heterogenicity can be seen within published studies on fetal loss following invasive testing, mainly due to the variable level of inclusion criteria, differences in study design and published outcome data on chorionicity. However, patients must be informed regarding the potential risks of invasive testing, particularly taking into consideration the factors that may increase rate of fetal loss such age maternal BMI, placental position and rate of baseline risk for fetal loss [216,217].

Additionally, fetal blood sampling (FBS) may be indicated for similar reasons as in singletons (e.g., fetal anemia, hydrops, congenital infections, thrombocytopenia). When performing FBS, the intrahepatic vein may be sampled to avoid confusing the cord origins in twins. The procedure-related loss rate is four-times higher than in singletons (8.2 vs 2.5%) [218].

Fetal Surveillance

The frequency of US evaluation in multiple pregnancy is determined by chorionicity. In DC pregnancies, surveillance is mainly directed at the detection of growth disorders. In MC pregnancies, surveillance is more frequent with additional Doppler measurements due to the higher risks of fetal demise and risk of complications specific to monochorionicity, as previously described. As discussed earlier, higher-risk multiple pregnancies should be cared for in a tertiary referral unit and for certain pregnancies this will require US monitoring performed in a fetal medicine centre.

DC Twin Pregnancy

There is a consensus among most international guidelines that DC twins should be scanned every four weeks, with more frequent assessments if any complications arise. The recommendation of ISUOG and NICE is that scans start at 24 weeks and occur every four weeks thereafter, with scans including fetal biometry (NICE recommend two or more biometric parameters) and AFV (NICE recommend using deepest vertical pocket (DVP)) and ISUOG recommend UA Doppler. Discordance in EFW should be calculated and recorded [54,92]. The ESPRiT multicentre prospective study assessed a two- versus a four-week US interval for detection of FGR and found that detection with a four-week interval reduced to 69% compared to 88% with a four-week interval [219].

Triplet Pregnancy

For trichorionic triamniotic triplet (TCTA) pregnancies, the frequency of surveillance is often increased with NICE recommending intervals of 14 days [54].

MC Pregnancy

The recommendation of NICE, RCOG, ISUOG and RANZCOG is that USs should be offered that monitor for TTTS, FGR and TAPS every 14 days from 16 weeks until birth. Scans should assess biometry, amniotic fluid in each sac and the UA PI (NICE recommend UA Doppler only in the presence of growth discordance or amniotic fluid discordance as does ACOG). The RCOG also highlights the importance of assessing the fetal bladders. There is variation in the recommendations related to MCA Dopplers, with ISUOG, RANZCOG and the International Federation of Gynecology and Obstetrics (FIGO) stating that these should be at every scan from 20 weeks and NICE and RCOG recommending that they are performed following laser therapy for TTTS or in the presence of sFGR [54,92,94, 154, 220,221].

A 2021 study by Nicholas et al. examined a series of international guidelines relating to management of MC pregnancies (25 guidelines). Conflicting recommendations were related to screening for TAPS, routine UA Doppler, umbilical vein and DV assessment. Published guidelines ranged from 2011 to 2020, revealing the necessity for many international guidelines to be updated with newly surfacing clinical work and ensuring a global consensus on the routine sonographic assessment of MC twins [113].

Growth Discordance and sFGR

A high index of suspicion is required to identify early signs of FGR and/or fetal growth discordance [94]. Both DC and MC twin pregnancies discordant for fetal growth are at higher risk of IUD compared with pregnancies with concordant BW. This is higher when at least one fetus is SGA [90]. As previously discussed, a discordance in CRL measurement in the first trimester of 20% or more is a risk factor for fetal growth disorders.

There is evidence that assessing EFW is less accurate in a twin than in a singleton pregnancy and ISUOG recommends the use of head, abdomen and femur measurements to calculate EFW, while NICE and RCOG recommend two or more biometric measurements from 16 weeks [54,92,94,222]. Singleton fetal growth charts are the most commonly used charts for plotting of EFW to aid growth surveillance and classification of SGA or FGR. There are differences in growth for twins compared to singletons in the third trimester and most marked in MC pregnancies with a slowing of growth in the third trimester. Thus, twin-specific growth charts have been developed and proposed [223,224]. However, it is not clear whether the mechanism behind this slowing of growth is pathological (i.e., FGR) or a physiological adaptation. There is observational evidence to suggest that the use of twin charts can reduce the rate of SGA diagnosis without compromising the detection of those fetuses at risk of adverse outcome [225]. However, singleton growth charts remain the gold standard at present. They provide the best predictors of adverse outcome in twins and may be used for evaluating growth abnormalities [226].

As discussed previously, a recommended cut-off of 20% difference between twins for discordance has been internationally adopted, given the increased risks of perinatal morbidity associated with a higher than 20% discordance [90]. For DC, MC and triplet pregnancies, NICE recommends that when discordance has been detected, increased monitoring with weekly UA Doppler is introduced when there is an EFW discordance of 20% or more and/or any of the babies has an EFW <10th centile for gestational age. The recommendation from ISUOG is UA Doppler every two weeks in DC with sFGR and weekly in MC pregnancies. When the EFW discordance is 25% or more and either baby has an EFW <10th centile then NICE recommends fetal medicine referral with ISUOG using the single indicator of discordance ≥25% and RCOG stating that this should occur in MC pregnancies when the discordance is ≥20% as the sole indicator [54,92,94]. Detection of a fetal weight discrepancy of 20% within the second trimester is recommended by ISUOG to prompt a detailed anatomical assessment, including screening for infection (cytomegalovirus, rubella and toxoplasmosis). Amniocentesis should also be considered [92].

Decisions relating to fetal surveillance, antenatal corticosteroid therapy and timing of delivery are normally driven by the smaller twin of a discordant pair. Heightened surveillance is indicated in those cases with an abnormal UA Doppler, including measurement of DV waveforms prior to 32–4 weeks. Amniotic fluid volume discordance is common, with the smaller twin showing a reduced DVP and the larger a mild increase. In MC twins, if the DVP is not <2 cm in the smaller and ≥8 cm before 20 weeks and ≥10 cm after 20 weeks in the larger, then this is discordant growth and liquor volumes and not TTTS [94]. However, this should always be considered a potential diagnosis (sometimes called 'pre-Stage 1 TTTS'), as TTTS may still develop.

Timing of delivery is challenging, and should consider chorionicity, gestational age at the time of growth discordance and Doppler abnormalities. One must also consider the added risks of prematurity for the normally grown co-twin. There is currently no RCT that explores different management options in twins with growth discordance. A 2022 IPD of 7,474 DCDA and 2,281 MC twin pairs derived from cohort studies demonstrated that growth discordance or SGA was associated with a higher absolute risk of stillbirth or NND. However, on balancing of these two risks, there was insufficient evidence to change the optimal timing for delivery based on the detection of growth disorders alone [227]. Decisions are often complex and require consistent parental counselling by a multidisciplinary team with significant expertise in managing multiple pregnancy with growth discordance [91].

For sFGR in DC pregnancies, ongoing management is as for singleton pregnancies with monitoring with UA, MCA and DV Doppler as appropriate [92]. However, the standard management of FGR requires modification in the case of twins, as the wellbeing of both twins needs to be considered. In the setting of sFGR in DC twins, decisions relating to timing of delivery are similar to those in singleton pregnancies, even if expectant management leads to the death of the smaller twin when delivery is delayed until a time when the risks of prematurity are acceptable for the appropriately grown twin.

For sFGR in a MC pregnancy, management and decisions are complicated by the heightened risk of co-twin demise or adverse neurological sequelae if one fetus dies, due to their shared circulation [91]. In MC pregnancies, the type and diameter of vascular anastomoses can influence outcome and give rise to different characteristics in the UA waveform. Thus, a classification system (Gratacos classification (Table 4)) based on UA Doppler waveforms in the smaller twin is now accepted [121]. These patterns are influenced by the flow across AA anastomoses: in type 1, 70% have large (>2 mm) anastomoses, with 18% in type 2 and 98% in type 3. There is an association with outcome (type 1 almost 100% survival, type 2 60% and type 3 85%, but sudden unpredictable demise in 15%, with 50% risk of death in larger co-twin): almost 100% of twin fetuses with type 1 sFGR survive, compared to 60% of those with type 2 [122]. Thus, UA Doppler studies from 24 weeks' gestation are recommended as standard care [94,228].

The management of severe growth discordance/sFGR in MC pregnancies is not currently established. Differences do exist compared to singleton pregnancies: for example, the latency that follows absent end-diastolic flow velocity before 'pre-terminal' factors ensue is longer in MC twins. Paradoxically, this reflects a temporary protective effect offered by the vascular anastomoses present in MC pregnancies. It is generally accepted that pregnancies with abnormal UA Doppler (sFGR types 2 and 3) should be assessed weekly, looking for signs of deterioration or progression to TTTS. If there are signs of imminent demise of the smaller twin (arrest of growth, anyhdramnios, abnormal venous Doppler) and delivery is not an option, then SR may be considered to protect the larger twin from the risks of co-twin demise or neurological disability (see Section 3.2.3). The course for type 3 sFGR is very unpredictable because the large placental anastomoses lead to large hemodynamic fluctuation [121]. This can lead to sudden acute transfusion events

Table 4 Classification system for selective intrauterine growth restriction in MC pregnancies according to UA Doppler flow in the smaller twin [121]

Classification system	Characteristics of UA Doppler flow during examination
Type 1	Positive end-diastolic flow in the UA
Type 2	Persistent absent or reversed end-diastolic flow
Type 3	Cyclical pattern of positive flow and absent or reversed end-diastolic flow

that are not predictable; therefore, antenatal testing cannot reliably predict demise. There is thus a significant risk of neurological damage in the non-growth-restricted fetus of 20–40% [229].

Pregnancies with type 1 sFGR should be monitored weekly with UA Doppler and middle cerebral artery (MCA) Doppler to exclude evolution of TAPS and are delivered electively at 34–6 weeks if there is satisfactory fetal growth velocity and normal UA waveforms. Type 1 sFGR is characterised by a good perinatal outcome when managed expectantly, and this represents the most reasonable management strategy for the large majority of affected cases [230]. In type 2 sFGR, as for type 3, delivery should be planned by 32 weeks, unless the fetal growth velocity is significantly abnormal or there is worsening of the fetal Dopplers [122]. Prenatal management of sFGR should be individualised according to gestational age at diagnosis, severity of growth discordance and magnitude of Doppler anomalies [231]. Options for intervention, other than delivery, are FLA and selective TOP in certain cases and are discussed further in Section 3.2.4.

New trials in this area are urgently needed, but in this rare and complex group, maximising the relevance and utility of clinical research design and outputs is paramount. In 2020, 11 core outcomes were formulated to facilitate standardised outcome collection and data reporting. These are live birth, gestational age at birth, BW, inter-twin BW discordance, death of surviving twin after death of co-twin, loss during pregnancy or before final hospital discharge, parental stress, procedure-related adverse maternal outcome, offspring length of hospital stay, neurological abnormalities on postnatal imaging, and childhood disability [232].

MCMA Twins

Currently there is little published evidence to advise on the most appropriate surveillance method for MCMA twins [233]. Management of MCMA pregnancies is similar to that of MCDA pregnancies, with careful assessment at the detailed anomaly scan and follow-up two-weekly for fetal biometry, fetal urinary bladder assessment, liquor volume and Doppler assessments from 24 to 26 weeks [107]. Frequent scanning is to identify early signs of MC-related complications including TTTS and discordance growth. In MCMA twins, 2020 data suggest BW discordance is not a sole indication for iatrogenic delivery, however, increased fetal monitoring is required due to the high association of growth discordance with fetal death [234]. The changes in UA Doppler parameters secondary to cord entanglement, including absent or end-diastolic flow and/or UA notching can occur intermittently or persistently in cases of MCMA twins. Previously, cord entanglement was thought to play a significant role, but data suggest that although this is almost invariably present at birth in MA twins, it is only implicated in causing fetal death before 24 weeks and thus if identified antenatally after 20 weeks can be expectantly managed with a good prognosis [117]. Furthermore, in those pregnancies where entanglement is present and perinatal mortality occurs after 24 weeks, other causes of death are now thought to be more relevant [118]. Monochorionic MA twins should be cared by fetal medicine specialists [233].

Prior literature has attempted to make recommendations on the choices between either continuous fetal monitoring as an elective inpatient within the third trimester or frequent outpatient monitoring (ranging from several times daily to alternate days) for MCMA twins, albeit displaying a degree of heterogenicity [235,236,237]. A 2019 systematic review of MCMA twins demonstrated an increased incidence of fetal loss during outpatient management versus inpatient management (7 vs 3%, respectively). However, the wide array of management protocols within the included studies and the varied gestational age at which the protocols were initiated may have resulted in an overall biased result [107].

The RCOG, ACOG, SMFM and NICE all advocate the delivery of MCMA twins by caesarean section between 32^{+0}- and 33^{+6}-weeks' gestation, following corticosteroid administration [54,94,154,155]. Following 32 weeks' gestation, 4 out of 100 MCMA pregnancies will result in fetal demise, whereas 1 out of 100 twins will die in the neonatal period because of prematurity [255]. Consequently, at this given gestational window, the risk of fetal demise outweighs the risk of prematurity, thus justifying the requirement for planned caesarean section prior to 34 weeks' gestation. Monochorionic MA twins are normally delivered by caesarean section due to the risk of intrapartum cord strangulation or the umbilical cord of the second twin becoming tethered around the first twin, risking cord transection and subsequent emergency caesarean section for the second twin [233].

SUMMARY OF MANAGEMENT OPTIONS

Prenatal Surveillance

Document dates and chorionicity: ideally this should be at 10–14 weeks or as soon as the multiple pregnancy is diagnosed after 14 weeks

- Confirm gestational age:
  - using the larger twin's CRL if 10–14 weeks
  - using a combination of HC, AC and femur length in combination after 14 weeks
  - in AR pregnancies, date by oocyte retrieval date +14 days.

(cont.)

- Document gestational sac position and fetal orientation (i.e., a lateral (left and right) or vertical (upper and lower)) should be utilised to accurately label twin pregnancies for ongoing fetal surveillance.
- Document chorionicity and amnionicity (though there is no prospective data to determine if this affects outcome).
- If transabdominal US scan views are poor because of a retroverted uterus or a high BMI, transvaginal US scan should be used to determine chorionicity and amnionicity.
- If chorionicity remains unconfirmed, manage as MC twins.
- MCMA twins and higher-order multiples should be referred to a tertiary fetal medicine centre for care by fetal medicine specialists.

Screening and Diagnosis of Fetal Abnormality

- Aneuploidy screening
  - Nuchal translucency (NT) screening alone provides fetus-specific risk.
  - The combined screening test (NT, β-hCG, PAPP-A) is recommended in twin pregnancies in the first trimester, though the accuracy is less than in singletons.
  - Offer second-trimester serum screening if a first-trimester screening unavailable or woman presents too late, however, detection rate is poor for multiple gestations.
  - Refer women with a risk of ≥1:150 to fetal medicine specialist in fetal medicine centre.
  - For higher-order multiples, only NT and maternal age can be used.
- Non-invasive prenatal testing using cffDNA, if available, should be offered after counselling as a contingent test.
- Perform a detailed anomaly US scan at 18^{+0}–20^{+6} weeks; this should include extended views of the heart. Be aware of increased risks of structural anomalies in MCMA pregnancies.
- Full fetal echocardiography is not routinely performed unless clinically indicated.
- Careful counselling about the increased risks of invasive diagnostic testing if indicated; it should be performed by an experienced operator in a tertiary fetal medicine centre with prior documentation of chorionicity,

(cont.)

fetal positions, placental site(s), septal site and location of cord insertions. For higher-order multiples, amniocentesis is the preferred option.

Fetal Surveillance

- In otherwise low-risk multiple pregnancies, fetal surveillance is determined by chorionicity.
- In MC twins (including MCMA), US evaluation should be performed every two weeks from 16 weeks' gestation. The US parameters that are recommended to record are
  - biometry
  - maximum pool depth of both sacs
  - umbilical artery Doppler from 24 weeks
  - assessment of bladder in both twins
  - recommendations for MCA Doppler vary.
- In low-risk DC twins, US evaluation is not standardised but is less frequent than for MC pregnancies and is commonly four-weekly from 20 weeks' gestation. The US parameters to be recorded are:
  - biometry
  - maximum pool depth of both sacs
  - recommendations for UA Doppler vary.
- There is no prospective data to show whether this increased surveillance improves outcome.
- In higher-order multiples, NICE recommends a frequency of every two weeks with the timing of initiation determined by chronicity as per twin pregnancies.
- Growth discordance and sFGR
  - a high index of suspicion is required
  - *first trimester:* CRL discrepancy of 20% or more should lead to 1) consideration of invasive testing for chromosomal abnormality and a detailed US scan in second trimester; if normal, 2) close surveillance of both twins for the pregnancy
  - *second and third trimester:* EFW should be calculated using at least two biometric measurements and the discordance in fetal weight calculated and recorded. Estimated fetal weight should be plotted on singleton growth charts
  - EFW discrepancy of 20% or more should lead to screening for viral infection, chromosomal and structural abnormality

(cont.)

- EFW discrepancy of 20% or more and/or EFW <10th centile should prompt increased surveillance comprising:
  - umbilical artery Doppler weekly
  - referral to fetal medicine if an MC pregnancy
- EFW of 25% or more and one or more fetus <10th centile should prompt a referral to fetal medicine for increased surveillance and management:
  - decisions regarding more detailed fetal surveillance (e.g., MCA and ductus venosus (DV) Doppler), corticosteroids and timing of delivery are complex and require the input and counselling of a multidisciplinary team.
- For sFGR in DC pregnancies, ongoing management is as for singleton pregnancies.
- For sFGR in MC pregnancies, the UA Doppler waveform helps classify the type of sFGR and guide management:
  - type 1 sFGR should have weekly surveillance and elective delivery at 34–6 weeks, if possible
  - types 2 and 3 sFGR should have weekly surveillance and elective delivery at 32 weeks, if possible.

3.2.4 Prenatal: Diagnosis and Management Options for Specific Complications

Multifetal Pregnancy Reduction

Multifetal pregnancy reduction (MFPR) is the termination of one or more normal embryos in a multifetal pregnancy to prevent higher-order pregnancies and the associated adverse outcomes [238]. This should be differentiated from selective termination, which involves the termination of an abnormal fetus. In certain settings, MFPR may be performed with the aim of reducing poor obstetric and perinatal outcomes. However, it should be noted that there is also a risk of early total pregnancy loss [239]. The acceptability of this is solely dependent upon a couple's social background, beliefs and wishes [240]. For most couples, MFPR is a more acceptable option than elective termination of the whole pregnancy.

The degree of procedural risk is dependent on the number of fetuses, chorionicity and gestational age at the time of the intervention. Reduction is usually performed at 11–14 weeks, as at this gestation the risk of spontaneous reduction or VTS has passed, and selection of the fetus may be based on first-trimester anomaly scan and NT [239]. A transabdominal percutaneous technique under US guidance is used, with the type of procedure determined by chorionicity and gestation. Intracardiac injection of potassium chloride, which is used to induce fetal asystole, can be employed in a singleton or member of a DC twin pair. In MC pregnancies, current management options include US-guided interstitial laser coagulation or radiofrequency ablation (RFA) up to around 22 weeks depending on fetal size, and bipolar cord coagulation between 18 and 25 weeks (sometimes later in a few centres). A 2015 meta-analysis between bipolar cord coagulation and RFA in MCDA demonstrated similar overall pooled survival rates of between 77 and 79% [241]. Within the first trimester, the choice of embryo to be reduced depends on multiple factors including anatomic features suggesting abnormality or aneuploidy (discordance in CRL, large NT), positioning of the embryo and operator dependent [239].

Reliable data regarding MFPR for quadruplets and above is lacking, however, it is well established that the rates of severe PTB, severe neonatal morbidity and indeed pregnancy loss are very high in these subsets of patients. It is therefore reasonable to assume that these risks will be lessened with MFPR.

For TCTA triplets, first-trimester intracardiac potassium chloride is the safest way to decrease the number of embryos present. However, a recent meta-analysis did not demonstrate a statistically significant reduction in the rate of miscarriage (<24 weeks) with MFPR in TCTA triplets compared to expectant management (7.4 vs 8.1%) [242]. The studies included were a small case series, which could have introduced substantial bias and heterogenicity, thus the results should be interpreted with caution. It should be noted that beyond 24 weeks, reduced triplet pregnancies (now DCDA twins) have a markedly lessened risk of PTB prior to 33 weeks (13.1%) compared to triplet pregnancies without intervention (35.1%) [243].

In DCTA triplets, whereby one part of the twins will be MC, the use of intracardiac potassium chloride, to either triplet (MCDA twin or singleton) has been noted to increase rates of pregnancy loss from 13.3 to 19.6% [244]. However, if successful, the rates of PTB substantially decreases regardless of whether the pregnancy is reduced to a singleton (46–8%) or to MCDA twins (46–23.1%) [240]. If intrafetal laser is used instead for DCTA triplets, thereby reducing the MCDA twin pair to a singleton, thus resulting in an overall DCDA twin pregnancy, the rate of miscarriage does not seem to change [244]. Conversely, the rate of co-twin death carries a significant risk of 12–46% depending on the modality used (RFA or laser, respectively) [245,246].

In triplet pregnancies without intervention, a 2009 systematic review reported that the risk of perinatal death was higher in DCTA than TCTA triplet pregnancies (OR: 3.3, 95% CI: 1.3–8.0), mainly owing to the higher risk of IUD in DCTA pregnancies (OR: 4.6, 95% CI: 1.8–11.7) [185]. The risk of neurological morbidity is also significantly higher in DCTA triplets (OR: 5.4, 95% CI: 1.6–18.3) [247]. Only one study has reported on outcomes of MC triamniotic (MCTA) pregnancies, and hence no formal comparison is possible. Reports do indicate that MFPR improves pregnancy outcome in triplet pregnancies regardless of initial fetal number, with reduced rates of pregnancy loss, antenatal complications, PTB, LBW and NND reported [240,242,247,248]. However, since no prospective randomised studies exist, and randomisation would prove exceptionally difficult in this setting, a couple's social background and beliefs remain pivotal to their informed decision-making process [249].

Although evidence is relatively limited, women undergoing MFPR commonly report immediate feelings of sadness and guilt. However, despite the significant emotional stress experienced, women appear to recover following reduction and overcome the psychological consequences. When making decisions regarding MFPR and selective termination, parents should be encouraged to weigh up the potential negative psychological impact against the risks and long-term consequences of pregnancy continuation [250].

Congenital Anomalies in Twins

In DC twins, the presence of a structural anomaly in one twin will not affect the healthy twin unless it is associated with polyhydramnios or spontaneous demise of the affected twin, thus increasing the risk of PTB with the risks of prematurity for the healthy twin. Careful consideration and counselling of parents must also occur when invasive procedures are being considered for the affected twin (e.g., shunt placement), as again these confer a risk of preterm delivery. For MC twins, the risk of spontaneous demise of the affected twin may have serious consequences for the healthy twin, with risks of massive hemodynamic changes and thus risk of death or cerebral damage to the healthy co-twin.

The management options for discordant anomalies are thus:

• conservative management
• selective termination of the affected twin
• termination of the whole pregnancy.

Prior to considering any intervention, chorionicity must be accurately determined, as the methods for selective feticide will differ. For DC twins, conservative management is usually the preferred option unless the wellbeing of the healthy twin is being compromised, to avoid the risk of procedure-related PTB, particularly if the anomaly is lethal. If the affected twin has a non-lethal anomaly but there is a significant risk of serious mental or physical disability, then parents need to be carefully counselled about the risks of intervention.

Selective Termination: Feticide

It is important to differentiate selective termination from MFPR. The former involves the presence of an abnormal fetus. In DC twins discordant for congenital anomaly, as discussed earlier, options include conservative management where the twin with the abnormality does not pose a risk to the healthy twin or selective termination in which feticide of the affected twin is performed. The latter may be performed by intracardiac or intrafunicular injection of potassium chloride or lidocaine once the affected twin has been carefully identified, as discussed earlier. Within the first trimester, the risk of pregnancy loss following the procedure is low, ranging from 2.1 to 5.8% [251]. Selective termination for fetal anomalies, whether chromosomal or structural, may occur at a later gestation (i.e., following a detailed anomaly scan at 18–22 weeks). Following identification of a fetal anomaly mid-trimester, many patients would opt for an immediate selective termination at this time, however, prior data of DCDA twins suggested this carries an increased risk of miscarriage (12–15%) or PTB of the healthy twin (>15%) [252]. As such, recommendations have been to postpone selective termination to 32 weeks' gestation, whereby severe PTB is mitigated, but it must be noted that once the procedure is undertaken at 32 weeks, approximately 45% of births will occur in the subsequent two weeks and there is a risk of spontaneous PTB whilst waiting for the procedure [239]. However, a meta-analysis of seven studies published in 2022, including 646 DC twins undergoing both early (<18 weeks' gestation) and late (>18 weeks' gestation) selective termination, demonstrated that the risk of pregnancy loss prior to 24 weeks was significantly lower in twin pregnancies undergoing early compared to late selective termination (1 vs 8%, OR: 0.25, 95% CI: 0.10–0.65, p = 0.004) [253]. The risk of PTB was significantly lower in DC twin pregnancies undergoing early compared to late selective termination when considering either PTB <37 weeks (19 vs 45%, OR: 0.36, 95% CI: 0.23–0.57, p <0.00001), <34 weeks (4 vs 19%, OR: 0.24, 95% CI: 0.11–0.54, p = 0.0005) and <32 weeks (3 vs 20%, OR: 0.21, 95% CI: 0.05–0.85, p = 0.03) [253]. The mean BW was also significantly greater in the early selective termination group (MD: 392.2 g; 95% CI: 59.1–726.7, p = 0.02). This highlights the importance of early diagnosis of fetal anomalies in twin pregnancies and subsequent consideration for prompt intervention rather than delay until the third trimester.

In MC twins, the procedure needs to be adapted to remove the risks to the healthy twin of transfer of the potassium chloride/lidocaine via placental anastomoses. This could lead to the subsequent death of the healthy twin. There are also risks of acute fetofetal haemorrhage with risk of mortality and morbidity either secondary to feticide or to death of the affected twin where conservative management is used. Thus, the technique employed must result not only in cardiac arrest, but isolation of the affected twin's circulation, and the techniques are like those employed in the TRAP sequence (see later) with the choice of procedure dependent on access and gestation. Given the risk of spontaneous demise of the affected twin, if selective feticide is to be undertaken in an MC pregnancy, it is preferable to perform this as soon as possible after diagnosis. Thus, in early gestation, intrafetal laser and RFA are the available options. In mid-gestation (18–25 weeks), RFA or bipolar energy are required to occlude the cord. At late gestation (>26 weeks), the size of the cord necessitates cord ligation. All procedures for selective feticide have risks, and the systematic review of procedures in MC twins by Gaerty et al. suggested that co-twin survival rates were highest with bipolar cord occlusion (84%) compared with RFA (73%); however, the incidence of PPROM occurred in 23% undergoing a bipolar cord occlusion, compared with just 11% in the RFA cohort [241]. In a 2021 study comparing outcomes of RFA prior to and after 16 weeks' gestation, there was no difference in the rate of co-twin loss (23.1 vs 29.7%, p = 0.558) or PPROM before 34 weeks (7.7 vs 5.4%, p = 0.853), or in the median gestational age at delivery (36.2 vs 37.3 weeks, p = 0.706) [254]. There is evidence that there may be a risk of adverse neurological sequelae in the surviving co-twin compared to that of an uncomplicated pregnancy [255]. Fetal magnetic resonance imaging (fMRI) four to six weeks post procedure for the surviving co-twin should be discussed.

In MCMA twins for severe discordant anomalies, selective feticide can be performed by US-guided bipolar cord coagulation and fetoscopic laser transection of the cord to allow disruption of cord entanglement, thus attempting to prevent demise of the healthy twin.

sFGR

When sFGR is severe in MC pregnancies and there are concerns regarding the in utero demise of the smaller twin, then intervention in the form of selective termination or FLA can be considered. While FLA of the vascular anastomoses is a proposed management option in type 2 and 3 cases, there is a significant risk of demise of the smaller twin (70%) and no difference in neurological outcome for survivors. In addition, it is technically very challenging owing to the reduction in amniotic fluid and the size of the anastomoses. For pregnancies complicated by type 2 or 3 sFGR, treatment with FLA also carries a high rate of mortality (44.3%) but low rate of morbidity compared with those managed expectantly, thereby supporting its use at gestations remote from neonatal viability [230]. Indications for selective termination include progressive deterioration in the condition of the smaller twin with evidence of significant risk of fetal demise (e.g., absent or reversed a-wave in the DV when delivery is not an option).

IUD of One Fetus (Single-Twin Demise, sIUFD)

A death of one twin may occur at any point during the antenatal period (single-twin demise or sIUFD), however, the time at which this occurs has a large influence on the prognosis for the co-twin [58,256,257]. When fetal death occurs in the first trimester, the evidence for the outlook for the co-twin is conflicting, with a 2021 paper stating there is little detrimental effect for the co-twin irrespective of chorionicity [258]. However, there have been reports of increased rates of PTB and SGA within the surviving twin.

In the second and third trimester, the risk of co-twin fetal demise is greater in MC twins. In a 2019 systematic review, MC pregnancies where sIUFD occurred at <28 weeks' gestation, the rate of co-twin IUD (OR: 2.31, 95% CI: 1.02–5.25) and NND (OR: 2.84, 95% CI: 1.18–6.77) significantly increased compared with sIUFD after 28 weeks' gestation [58]. The overall rates of co-twin fetal demise were doubled in MC twins compared to DC twins with rates of abnormal postnatal brain imaging at a six-fold increase in MC twins [58].

Healy et al. published in 2022 a proposed management plan, based on expert consensus for sIUFD [259]. Once a diagnosis of fetal demise has been confirmed, immediate assessment of fetal wellbeing of the co-twin should commence, including fetal biometry, liquor volume assessment, Doppler velocimetry and placental examination, irrespective of chorionicity [259]. Women and their partners should be counselled on the prognosis of current findings and chorionicity and referral to bereavement services should be offered. For DC twins, two- to four-weekly US and Doppler velocimetry assessments should take place until delivery. It is recommended that MC twins undergo more frequent Doppler velocimetry assessments, with weekly DV, UA and fetal cerebral measurements for the first four weeks and then fortnightly thereafter [259]. This includes measuring MCA peak systolic velocity (PSV) to look for evidence of fetal anemia. If detected prior to 35 weeks in MC twins, intrauterine transfusion (IUT) is advised. For MC twins, fMRI of the surviving co-twin can be offered, however, timing of this investigation should be timed to provide information prior to birth, accepting that brain injury may not be detectable initially [259].

A major challenge is the decision regarding timing of delivery, as the risk of the co-twin dying must be balanced against preterm-associated morbidity and mortality, secondary to iatrogenic preterm delivery. International consensus (RCOG, ISUOG, RANZCOG, NICE, FIGO), Society Obstetricians and Gynecologists of Canada (SOGC) and ACOG) recommend the avoidance of preterm delivery for the surviving twin [54,83,92,94,154,155,200,221]. For DC twins, this is recommended between 37^{+0} and 37^{+6} weeks' gestation, however, for MC twins, delivery should be considered by 36^{+6} weeks [83]. The timing should be individualised for the parents, taking into account the assessment findings and the couple's views and wishes and their past obstetric history. The mode of delivery should also be discussed thoroughly with the patient and partner. Whilst there is no absolute contraindication for either vaginal delivery or caesarean section, it should be noted that recent literature has demonstrated a statistically significant increase rate of emergency caesarean if sIUFD occurred in the presenting twin (67 vs 32%, OR: 4.29, 95% CI: 1.25–14.7, p = 0.02) [260].

After birth, a thorough neonatal examination should be performed including neurological investigation and the value of a post-mortem examination of the dead twin should be discussed with the parents. The placenta should undergo investigation and confirmation of chorionicity. Ideally, the survivor should be enrolled in long-term neurological and developmental follow-up, alongside postnatal magnetic resonance imaging (MRI) brain imaging. There is a need for core outcome sets for the assessment of sIUFD in twin pregnancies [58,81].

TRAP Sequence

The diagnosis of TRAP is reliably made on US in the first trimester, when the condition is characterised by an abnormal fetus that has no functional cardiac activity but may show movements and grow. Doppler studies demonstrate the pathognomonic features of reversed arterial perfusion through an AA anastomosis. The goal of management in TRAP is to maximise the fetal outcome for the pump twin; however, at present, there is currently no clear guideline on the management of TRAP when deciding on choice of intervention. Options for management include the conservative approach with serial sonographic assessment or intervention to arrest the circulation of the acardiac twin. At diagnosis, biometric measurements of the acardiac twin should be taken and an assessment of the structures present, liquor volume and features of cardiac failure in the pump twin made. An acardiac/pump weight ratio >70% has been associated with poor prognosis. However, it must be noted that normal biometric measurements may not be possible in the acardiac twin and thus rapid growth of the acardiac twin (using length) can also be used as a criterion [261]. In the absence of polyhydramnios and signs of cardiac failure, conservative management may be appropriate with serial US to look for development of these features, and to monitor the growth of the acardiac twin. There are currently no RCTs examining conservative management versus intervention for TRAP patients; however, a recent systematic review by Mone et al. demonstrated better survival with intervention than with conservative management (OR: 2.22, 95% CI: 1.23–4.01, p = 0.008), but again confirmed that this difference was greater in the presence of one or more poor prognostic features (OR: 8.58, 95% CI: 1.47–49.96, p = 0.02). There was insufficient data to determine which poor prognostic features should guide management [262].

The type of interventional procedure performed will depend on the clinical presentation and gestation. Options include coagulation of umbilical cord and/or placental anastomoses, intrafetal laser or RFA, and these can be offered at the time of diagnosis or around 16 weeks' gestation if there has been no spontaneous cessation of flow. Radiofrequency ablation has been the most common intervention reported within the literature, with most studies retrospectively examining cohorts of MC twins. However, studies have included the treatment of RFA for multiple additional pathologies (TTTS, sFGR) and not just TRAP. The literature since 2020 has suggested an overall survival rate of approximately 70–80%, with gestational age at delivery ranging from 34 to 37 weeks [254,263,264,265,266]. Bipolar cord coagulation can also be used to treat TRAP, however, available reporting literature on this modality is sparser than RFA. Overall co-twin survival has been reported to range between 55 and 63%, with gestational age at delivery at around 31 weeks [267,268]. A 2022 meta-analysis of eight studies examining RFA versus bipolar cord coagulation demonstrated lower rates of PPROM (OR: 0.45, 95% CI: 0.27–0.73), longer procedure to delivery intervals (mean difference: 13.42 days, 95% CI: 1.90–24.94) and less PTB (OR: 0.50, 95% CI: 0.29–0.85) following RFA [269]. There is limited data on the efficacy of intrafetal laser for the treatment of TRAP, however, the same 2022 paper reported a metanalysis of three studies that did not show any difference in overall survival or gestational age at delivery when comparing intrafetal laser and RFA [269]. Microwave ablation (MWA) is an additional interventional modality with promising future application. A 2019 paper reported a 73% survival rate with a median delivery gestation of 37.6 weeks [270]. In conjunction, Xie et al. are currently piloting an RCT comparing MWA versus RFA, which may provide promising results on this relatively new treatment modality and its application within the context of TRAP [271].

The decision on when to intervene has also been discussed in the literature. Most published studies (including the ones cited earlier) examining interventional therapy for TRAP are from 16 weeks' gestation and above. However, several studies have aimed to elucidate whether intervention before 16 weeks has clinical benefit. A small series of 12 cases undergoing intrafetal laser at a median gestational age of 13^{+5} weeks demonstrated an overall survival of 91.7% and only a single case of PTB [272]. Weber et al. in 2021 evaluated 15 MA pregnancies with TRAP diagnosed before 14 weeks' gestation and compared expectant management to intrafetal laser [273]. All pump twins that had expectant management died before 20 weeks while 57% of pump twins in the intervention group survived with a median gestational age at delivery of 39.6 weeks [273]. With these results taken collectively, intrafetal laser therapy may hold promise as the main treatment intervention for TRAP within the first or early second trimester. However, the studies included are of very small sample sizes, with high risk of publication bias. An ongoing RCT, the 'TRAP Intervention Study: early versus late intervention for twin reversed arterial perfusion sequence', is aimed at addressing this important question on gestational age of intervention [274]. Results of this study may provide key novel insights on optimal timing of intervention.

TTTS

The pathophysiology of TTTS is not fully understood, and although vascular anastomoses are a prerequisite for its development, there is no unique pattern. The chronic imbalance in net flow leads to hypovolemia, oliguria and oligohydramnios in the donor and hypervolemia, polyuria and polyhydramnios in the recipient, who may also develop circulatory overload and hydrops. Cordocentesis studies demonstrate that 75% of cases will have an inter-twin haemoglobin difference <15%, and thus the syndrome is not simply due to transfer of red blood cells [275]. Discordant growth, with the recipient being larger and the donor being small, is usually present but not essential. There may be signs of right ventricular dysfunction in the recipient, and specialists consider presence of tricuspid regurgitation to be an abnormal Doppler waveform and a marker of severity. These features must be carefully documented before and after any intervention and counselling individualised to reflect the whole clinical picture. Endocrine factors, related to fluid and pressure homeostasis, are likely to contribute to the varying degrees of clinical severity.

A TTTS diagnosis is made when the following US criteria are seen:

- a single placental mass
- concordant gender

- oligohydramnios with maximum vertical pocket (DVP) <2 cm in one sac and polyhydramnios with DVP ≥8 cm (>10 cm after 20 weeks) in the other sac (Figure 5).

A spectrum of TTTS exists, ranging from mild disease with isolated discordant AFV, to severe disease with demise of one or both twins. The Quintero staging system aids standardisation of TTTS, using five stages, as outlined in Table 5 [124]. However, since TTTS does not often progress in a predictable manner and the staging is not strongly predictive of outcome, its clinical utility has been questioned. Atypical TTTS has been noted in approximately 7% of cases, whereby cardiac compromise or abnormal Dopplers can be noted in either twin prior to the alteration of AFV that meets the desired cut-off [276]. The RCOG suggests that structural and/or functional assessment of the fetal

Table 5 Quintero staging system for TTTS [124]

Stage I	The bladder of the donor twin is still visible, and Doppler studies are normal
Stage II	The bladder of the donor twin is not visible, but Doppler studies are not critically abnormal
Stage III	Doppler studies are critically abnormal in either twin (UA in donor and/or DV in recipient); absent or reverse end-diastolic velocity in the UA, reverse flow in the DV or pulsatile umbilical venous flow
Stage IV	Recipient hydrops; ascites, pericardial or pleural effusion, scalp oedema or overt hydrops
Stage V	Intrauterine demise of one or both twins

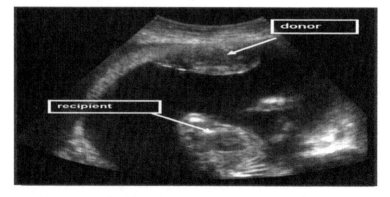

Figure 5 US imaging in TTTS, showing donor and recipient

heart (especially in the recipient) by echocardiography may be useful in defining the prognostic risk of severe TTTS and treatment modalities [94]. Quintero stages I and II have a significant proportion of recipient twins with ventricular hypertrophy, atrioventricular valve regurgitation and objective abnormalities in either right or left ventricular function. Discordant bladder appearances and/or evidence of hemodynamic and cardiac compromise are strongly indicative of severe disease [94].

Strict AFV cut off values have been recommended by the Eurofetus group. However, a 2021 paper reporting 366 TTTS cases between 20 and 26 weeks' gestation found 14.5% of patients might be excluded from laser treatment if the MVP for the recipient twin is confined to ≥10 cm [277]. It can be noted that 60.4% of these patients were Quintero stage III or IV. Between gestation weeks 16 and 17, a DVP of amniotic fluid measuring 7 cm equates to the 97.5th centile. Consequently, Khalil et al. suggested modifying the DVP cut-off prior to 18 weeks from 8 to 6 cm to avoid misdiagnosis and postponement of TTTS, thus potentially reducing the number of poor outcomes resulting from delaying intervention [278,279]. However, complete laser coagulation of the vascular equator for an anterior placenta with a DVP <8 cm may prove more challenging or even impossible.

Several first-trimester markers have been investigated for prediction of development of FFTS, including NT discordance or NT >95th centile, CRL discordance and reversed a-wave in the DV on Doppler study. None of these individually predicts the development of TTTS with sufficient accuracy, and thus combinations of tests and the addition of biomarkers are being studied in the research setting [202]. The current practice is to use regular US surveillance.

Recent developments in prenatal care strategies and management options for patients with TTTS have reduced perinatal mortality rates significantly. Left untreated, TTTS is associated with severe complications, and despite therapy, neonatal mortality and morbidity remain high [280]. Treatment options for TTTS include expectant management, amnioreduction, septostomy, FLA of vascular anastomoses (Figure 6) and SR. The two main options are serial amniodrainage (percutaneous insertion of a needle into the recipient sac to remove amniotic fluid and to bring DVP back to normal limits) and FLA with amniodrainage. The aim of FLA is to disconnect the two fetal circulations. A Cochrane review comparing randomised and quasi-randomised studies of septostomy, amnioreduction and FLA included three studies (253 women and 506 babies) [281]. There was no difference in overall death rate between amnioreduction and FLA (average RR: 0.87, 95% CI: 0.55–1.38 adjusted for clustering, two trials), or death of at least one infant per pregnancy (RR: 0.91, 95% CI: 0.75–1.09, two trials), or death of both infants per pregnancy (average

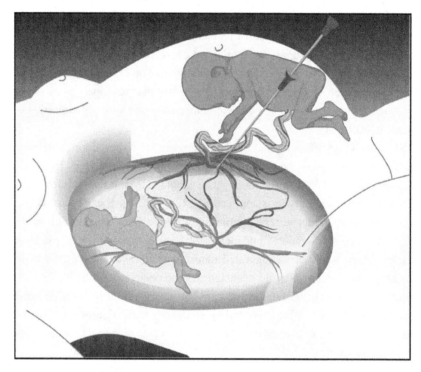

Figure 6 FLA. After El Kateb, A, Ville, Y. Update on twin-to-twin transfusion syndrome. Best Pract Res Clin Obstet Gynaecol. 2008; 22(1): 63–75

RR: 0.76, 95% CI: 0.27–2.10, two trials) [282,283]. It should be noted that for the outcomes of death, the two included trials demonstrated opposite effects, with the Eurofetus trial demonstrating a reduction in mortality with FLA, and the National Institute of Child Health and Human Development trial (NIHCD) demonstrating a reduction with amnioreduction, although for this result the CIs crossed the line of no effect. This may partly reflect that in the NIHCD trial all cases underwent amnioreduction prior to randomisation, which may have affected outcome, and the trial was stopped early. However, long-term studies found more babies were alive without neurological abnormality at the age of six years in the laser group than in the amnioreduction groups (RR: 1.57, 95% CI: 1.05–2.34 adjusted for clustering, Eurofetus trial) [282]. It must also be recognised that the majority of pregnancies in the included trials were Quintero stage II or III (three stage IV in the Eurofetus trial and three in NIHCD) and were less than 26 weeks' gestation, limiting the applicability of the results to this population. However, in light of the review findings, FLA is recommended first-line for management of TTTS and is consequently endorsed by RCOG, SMFM, ISUOG and RANZCOG [92,94,155,220].

The management of stage I TTTS remains controversial. Systematic reviews have demonstrated progression occurs in 27% of pregnancies and survival rates for at least one twin were 85, 87 and 92% if managed expectantly, by laser or amnioreduction, respectively [284,285]. An international RCT compared cases of stage I FFTS that were managed conservatively (n = 58) versus immediate laser treatment (n = 59). Of the cases managed conservatively, 59% progressed (n = 34) and required rescue laser therapy. However, the overall survival rates were of no significant difference between each original group (77 and 78%, respectively) [286]. As such, expectant management with regular fetal US surveillance is a reasonable option and many fetal medicine centres adopt this line of practice [286]. It allows for a proportion of patients to avoid unnecessary intervention, which in itself can carry a risk of poor outcome. However, given the unpredictability of stage I TTTS, in depth counselling of patients regarding patient wishes and potential outcomes is paramount [112]. Wohlmuth et al. postulated the incorporation of early sonographic cardiovascular markers, including inter-twin DV time-interval differences (preload) and aortic distention (afterload), rather than the present or absence of bladder filling to assist in selecting patients that may benefit from early FLA treatment in stage I disease [282]. It was noted that such cardiac changes may even precede the identification of stage I TTTS by on average 12±6 days [287]. However, the benefit of these parameters is yet to be studied in large multicentre RCTs.

Regarding the degree of TTTS severity, the Quintero staging has been the longstanding diagnostic tool for MC twins. However, as survival rates following laser therapy have continued to improve, its use in predicting prognosis is questioned. A 2020 systematic review assessed 20 studies for outcomes for pregnancies complicated by TTTS according to Quintero stage and found that overall survival was higher for stage I and II but rates were moderately high for III and IV when FLA is performed. Gestational age at birth was similar for stages I–III [285]. A 2022 systematic review assessed 10 studies (4,031 fetuses with TTTS) and found that donor demise was associated with high Quintero stages compared with surviving donors (OR: 2.42, 95% CI: 1.78–3.29, p <0.001, I^2 = 0%). Recipient fetal demise had a trend for higher Quintero stage compared with surviving recipients, but the analysis did not achieve statistical significance. Pregnancies with donor demise had lower gestational at the time of FLA (mean difference: −0.56, 95% CI: −0.93 to −0.18, p = 0.003, I^2 = 36%), whereas pregnancies complicated by recipient demise had similar gestational at time of FLA compared with those without demise [288].

Monochorionic MA twins complicated by TTTS are at even greater risk of perinatal mortality. A 2020 systematic review of 15 cohort studies including 888 MCMA twins, of which 44 were complicated by TTTS, compared interventional outcomes between FLA and amnioreduction [289]. In cases treated by laser surgery, the incidence of miscarriage, IUD, NND and postnatal death was 19.6, 27.4, 7.4 and 35.9%, respectively. In cases treated with amniodrainage, the incidence of IUD, NND and perinatal death was 31.3, 13.5 and 45.7% respectively [289]. Thus, survival rates are lower in MCMA twins, however, FLA still remains the favourable management choice for this subset of MC twins. Given the associated morbidity, termination of the whole pregnancy should always be considered as a management option.

Fetoscopic laser ablation is performed percutaneously under local or regional anaesthesia. A cannula or fetoscopic sheath is inserted into the amniotic sac and the placenta inspected. The arterio-venous (AV) anastomoses are identified, and the laser tip directed at a 90° angle and the vessel photocoagulated (selective technique). Following the laser treatment, amniodrainage is performed to a normal DVP value. Residual anastomoses are reported in up to 33% of treated pregnancies, and these can lead to complications such as TAPS (13%) and recurrent TTTS (14%) [290]. The Solomon technique was thus proposed, involving coagulation of the whole vascular equator, ensuring to include tiny non-visualised anastomoses [291].

In an RCT of 274 patients, comparing both techniques against each other, the Solomon technique was associated with fewer cases of recurrent TTTS (1 vs 7%) and additional post-laser TAPS (3 vs 16%) [292]. A subsequent two-year follow-up of the original cohorts did not display any significant differences in either group regarding neurodevelopmental outcomes or neonatal morbidity [293]. A systematic review comparing Solomon versus the selective technique (three studies, n = 523) has demonstrated a trend towards a reduction in recurrent TTTS and TAPS and an increase in twin survival with no increase in complications or adverse events [294]. In 2021, Kanazawa et al. examined the rate of placental abruption and PPROM following either the selective (n = 227) or Solomon (n=168) technique for the treatment of TTTS. The incidences of placental abruption (Solomon vs selective: 10.7 vs 3.5%, p = 0.007) and PPROM with subsequent delivery before 32 weeks (20.2 vs 7.1%, p <0.01) were higher in the Solomon group. However, the rate of at least one surviving twin was significantly higher after Solomon's laser surgery (98.2 vs 93.8%, p = 0.046) [295]. Increasing rates of placental abruption following the Solomon technique were also detected recently by Knijnenburg et al. in a large retrospective cohort study, however, results were not significantly different (OR: 0.50, 95% CI: 0.18–1.39, p = 0.184) [296]. It is theorised that higher rates of placental abruption following the Solomon method are due to the larger volume of placental tissue that is ablated, including normal healthy placental tissue. As such, many clinicians opt for a partial Solomon technique, ablating areas of neighbouring anastomoses around the vascular equator, but aiming not to damage any areas of healthy placental tissue [112]. Reported maternal complications following TTTS include nausea, vomiting and abdominal pain presumed to be due to secondary leakage of amniotic fluid into the peritoneal cavity [297].

Whilst the type of technique for laser therapy may risk PTB, CL at the time of treatment has a significant association with subsequent risk [298,299,300]. Buskmiller et al. retrospectively analysed cases of patients with short cervixes that underwent a variety or treatments prior to laser therapy from 2011 to 2020 [301]. Patients with a short cervix (<30 mm) with FFTS were managed either expectantly (59%), with vaginal progesterone (13%), with pessary insertion (8%), with cerclage placement (8%) or with a combination of treatments (30%) [301]. It was noted that the use of interventions for a short cervix prior to laser surgery were of no increased superiority when prolonging pregnancy compared with managing cases expectantly. However, the retrospective nature of this study introduced a large risk of bias and definitions of a short cervix remain inconsistent. Well-designed RCTs are required to determine the true efficacy of each therapy for short cervix specifically within this context.

Centres performing FLA should have adequate training and experience and continued throughout to maximise perinatal survival and minimise perinatal morbidity, and outcomes (and operator performance) should be prospectively audited [297]. Even after 'successful therapy', the fetuses remain high risk and require careful US surveillance both for the occurrence of complications (e.g., recurrent TTTS, limb defects) and for the assessment of fetal cardiac function and brain anomalies. An fMRI of the fetal brain is recommended four weeks after surgery to assess for brain injury. The recommendations for timing of delivery in TTTS cases have not yet been fully established. Many experts advocate premature elective delivery of such babies between 34 and 36 weeks. However, in the absence of any post-laser complications, the 2022 literature has recommended delivery between 36^{+0} and 37^{+0} gestational weeks [112].

Twin-to-twin transfusion syndrome can occur with MA twins but is less common due to the protective large bidirectional AA anastomoses, thus is seen in 2–4% of MCMA pregnancies. The diagnosis is made by the presence of polyhydramnios in the single sac with a small or invisible bladder in one twin and a distended bladder in the other. The best treatment option is unclear, as FLA is often more challenging and with greater risks due to the proximity of the cord insertions and overlapping vascular territories [117]. A systematic review reported 44 cases of TTTS in MCMA pregnancies with conservative management having a 60% neonatal survival, laser 48% and cord occlusion 80% [289].

TAPS

Twin anemia-polycythemia sequence develops in the absence of the severe oligo-hydramnios–polyhydramnios sequence needed for a diagnosis of TTTS, although mild discordance of liquor volumes may be present, as may growth discordance. It can occur across a wide range of gestation from 15 to 35 weeks but is more commonly seen in later pregnancy and can be spontaneous (5%) or occur after FLA for TTTS (2–16%) [302]. It is characterised by a large haemoglobin discrepancy between the twins, with anemia in the donor twin and polycythemia in the recipient twin (predicted antenatally by Doppler US MCA-PSV assessment). Current clinical cut-off values are generally elevated MCA-PSV >1.5 MoM in the donor and decreased MCA-PSV <1.0 MoM in the recipient. However, more recent research identified that a difference of >0.375 MCA-PSV MoM is likely to already predict haemoglobin discordance between twins greater than the 95th percentile and an inter-twin difference in MCA-PSV >0.5 MoM is a more superior predictor of TAPS, irrespective of absolute Doppler velocities [303,304]. As a result, a 2020 Delphi consensus recommends the addition of an MCA-PSV discordance of ≥1.0 MoM to the existing definitions of MCA-PSV ≥1.5 MoM in the donor twin and ≤0.8 MoM for the recipient twin [305]. Co-existing FGR commonly occurs in TAPS pregnancies and usually affects the donor [302]. A prenatal classification system for TAPS exists with stages 1–5; stages 1–2 are differences in MCA-PSV without signs of fetal compromise, stage 3 is with cardiac compromise of the donor, stage 4 hydrops and stage 5 IUD [303].

Screening for TAPS is controversial, with increasing discussion internationally around routine screening in all MC twins. There is currently a lack of evidence to demonstrate that screening improves outcomes, with no clear treatment pathway and no health economic evidence, and thus current NICE guidance does not advocate screening in all MC twins. Screening in complicated MC pregnancies (post FLA for TTTS and sFGR) is advocated [54].

Postnatally, diagnosis requires an inter-twin haemoglobin difference of 80 g/l (8 g/dl) with a demonstrable chronic transfusion imbalance (placenta with small anastomoses or donor/recipient reticulocyte count ratio >1.7) [306]. Placentas from both spontaneous and iatrogenic TAPS are very similar, typically showing 3–4 small (≤1 mm) unidirectional AV anastomoses with the paucity of compensatory AA anastomoses, unlike TTTS, where there are large central diameter AV anastomoses [306,307]. Compensatory AV anastomoses can however be seen in 10–19% of spontaneous TAPS, compared to 25% of TTTS placentas [306]. The development of small unidirectional vascular connections without compensatory vascular networks is presumed to increase the chronic net transfer of red blood cells, leading to the development of TAPS [306,308].

Complications of TAPS include severe anemia leading to hydrops in the donor, and severe polycythemia in the recipient that may lead to cardiac failure and cerebral vascular accidents. Both twins are at risk of later IUD. Once a TAPS diagnosis has been made, the management options available are dependent on gestational age, etiology of TAPS (spontaneous or post-operatively), accessibility of the placental vascular equator and severity of the condition [303].

Where elective delivery is not an option, expectant management with close weekly US monitoring (including MCA-PSV measurements) or supportive interventions, which encompasses cordocentesis and IUT, may be utilised in the first instance. The expectant approach is favoured in TAPS cases that present in the first or early second trimesters, as many cases may remain stable, by which the goal of a late preterm delivery can feasibly be achieved. More invasive management options include an IUT of the anemic donor twin or an exchange transfusion whereby blood from the recipient twin is removed and transfused to the donor twin [309]. If there is rapid recurrence of the anemia after two transfusions then options again include elective delivery if at an appropriate gestational age and EFW, or selective feticide or FLA of the vascular anastomoses depending on gestation, fetal condition and accessibility of the equator. It is however imperative to avoid transfusions in cases of severe TAPS given the rapid inter-twin passage of blood, which may risk transfer of blood to the polycythemia recipient, leading to worsening hyperviscosity [125]. Intraperitoneal transfusion of fetal blood can assist in mitigating this risk factor, allowing for slower red cell absorption by the donor and reduce hyperviscosity of the recipient [310].

At present, FLA is the only potentially curative in utero treatment for TAPS. However, this is more technically challenging than in the context of TTTS. The presence of a floating inter-twin membrane can inhibit the ability to fully visualise the vascular equator and any small vessels requiring ablation [303]. Performing an FLA for TAPS that occurs after FLA for TTTS will have the added complication of this being a second procedure and thus knowledge of the first procedure and any challenges (e.g., blood-stained liquor) can inform the decision as to whether to perform a repeat laser for TAPS.

There is currently no consensus as to the best management for TAPS. Data from the TAPS registry, across 17 fetal medicine centres, demonstrated that of 370 cases recorded, 31% were managed expectantly, 30% with laser surgery and 19% with IUT. A small proportion were managed with delivery or selective feticide (8 and 1%, respectively). Perinatal mortality was high across all groups (mortality: 17% expectant, 18% laser, 18% IUT, 10% delivery and 7% co-twin following feticide). There was also significant morbidity (49% delivery group,

31% laser, 25% selective feticide, 31% expectant). The longest diagnosis to birth internal was in the selective feticide group followed by laser surgery, expectant and delivery [311]. For patients presenting prior to 28 gestational weeks, recent literature has suggested an operative approach, with laser surgery ensuring a greater proportion of patients are resolved of TAPS prior to delivery, alongside delivering at an adequate gestational age [312].

The data from the TAPS registry was included in a 2021 meta-analysis of 38 studies (506 pregnancies) assessing the perinatal outcome according to whether TAPS occurred spontaneously or post laser treatment, whilst examining the outcome following each management option. Intrauterine death occurred in 5.2% (95% CI: 3.6–7.1%) of twins with spontaneous TAPS and in 10.2% (95% CI: 7.4–13.3%) of those with post-laser TAPS, while the corresponding rates of NND were 4.0% (95% CI: 2.6–5.7%) and 9.2% (95% CI: 6.6–12.3%), respectively [298]. Overall, IUD occurred in 9.8% (95% CI: 4.3–17.1%) of twins managed expectantly and in 13.1% (95% CI: 9.2–17.6%), 12.1% (95% CI, 7.7–17.3%) and 7.6% (95% CI, 1.3–18.5%) of those treated with laser surgery, IUT and SR, respectively [298]. Severe neonatal morbidity affected 27.3% (95% CI: 13.6–43.6%) of twins in the expectant-management group, 28.7% (95% CI: 22.7–35.1%) of those in the laser-surgery group, 38.2% (95% CI: 18.3–60.5%) of those in the IUT group and 23.3% (95% CI: 10.5–39.2%) of those in the SR group [313]. Results of this review suggest that twins complicated by spontaneous TAPS may have a better prognosis. The TAPS trial, a multicentre open label RCT is currently underway to evaluate the effect of laser surgery compared with standard treatment on the neonatal outcome and gestational age of delivery in MC twin gestations complicated by TAPS [314]. It is hoped that completion of this study will be in 2024.

Postpartum, the outcomes of TAPS can range from haematological disorders to severe neonatal morbidity and mortality. Postnatal TAPS can manifest as anemia in the donor twin, polycythemia in the recipient [128]. The discordance in haemoglobin may warrant a blood transfusion within the donor twin, with partial exchange in the recipient twin to minimise hyperviscocity-related complications [303]. Thrombocytopenia can also develop postnatally, more commonly in the recipient twin. Postnatal TAPS tends to be seen less frequently in cases managed by laser therapy, compared with cases managed expectantly. Neonatal morbidity or cerebral injury can range from 25 to 49% of TAPS cases [303,311,312]. A retrospective study published in 2020 examined the long-term neurological sequalae of survivors of spontaneous TAPS cases. Ex-donors were noted to have an up to 15% rate of deafness and a four-fold increase in neurodevelopmental impairment. This was a significant increase compared to ex-recipients (OR: 4.1, 95% CI: 1.8–9.1, p = 0.001) [315]. Ultimately, regardless of the management option, the importance of minimising risk of prematurity and residual morbidity of TAPS cases is paramount for the overall long-term neurological benefit and neonatal survival.

Conjoined Twins

Owing to the very poor prognosis for all types of conjoined twins, with no in utero fetal interventions possible, TOP should be discussed. Conjoined twins are rare, and prenatal assessment is required in a tertiary centre so that diagnosis can be confirmed, and prognosis discussed in conjunction with a multidisciplinary team, as advised by RCOG [94].

If the parents decide to continue with the pregnancy, then a detailed US examination including echocardiogram should be performed, with consideration of other imaging modalities such as 3D US and fMRI [316]. The aim of imaging is to determine the amount of shared tissue and organ involvement, particularly cardiac, as this has the greatest influence on mortality and the ability to separate the twins. If preterm labour occurs, then vaginal delivery can be considered, but for most, caesarean section is required as dystocia is common [317]. Delivery should be carefully planned in a tertiary centre with appropriate neonatal and paediatric surgical support [318].

SUMMARY OF MANAGEMENT OPTIONS

Prenatal: Diagnosis and Management Options for Specific Complications

MFPR

- Multifetal pregnancy reduction aims to reduce poor obstetric and perinatal outcomes associated with higher-order pregnancies.
- Acceptability is dependent upon couple's social background, beliefs and wishes.
- In DC twins, the preferred method is US-guided intracardiac potassium chloride injection.
- In MC pregnancies, options are US-guided interstitial laser coagulation or RFA at <18 weeks or bipolar cord coagulation at 18–25 weeks.
- Multifetal pregnancy reduction of triplet pregnancy remains contentious; studies of MFPR of quadruplets and higher-order pregnancies are lacking.
- Anti-D prophylaxis is required for procedures.

Congenital Anomalies in Twins

- For all twins:
  - offer counselling and psychological support

(cont.)
- accurate chorionicity determination is essential
- anti-D prophylaxis is required for procedures
- options:
  - conservative management
  - selective feticide of the abnormal fetus
  - termination of the pregnancy

- Dichorionic twins:
  - conservative management is usually preferred if the condition is lethal to avoid intervention loss rates
  - selective feticide, if indicated, can be performed at a later gestation (i.e., following the detailed anomaly scan at 20–2 weeks)
- Monochorionic twins:
  - conditions with a high risk of intrauterine fetal death selective feticide should be considered
- Careful follow-up of surviving normal twin

Selective Termination: Feticide

- In DZ twins, use intracardiac or intrafunicular injection of potassium chloride or lidocaine.
- Counselling couples with DZ twins: inform them that delivery of a viable infant/s is most often achieved, but complications include miscarriage and preterm delivery. Gestational age at feticide does not significantly affect miscarriage rates.
- In MC pregnancies, selective feticide is to be undertaken as soon as possible after diagnosis and options are US-guided interstitial laser coagulation or RFA at <18–25 weeks, bipolar cord coagulation at 18–25 weeks and cord ligation from 26 weeks; co-twin survival rates and preterm rupture of membrane rates vary with the procedure used.
- In MCMA pregnancies, bipolar cord coagulation and fetoscopic laser transection of the cord can be used.
- In MC pregnancies, fMRI should be discussed with the parents to assess for neurological sequalae in the surviving co-twin.
- Psychological support of parents is important before and after feticide.

(cont.)
sFGR

- Management options are expectant, FLA, selective termination or delivery at later gestations. The role of FLA is not clear.

IUD of One Fetus (Single Twin Demise, sIUFD)

- For all twins:
  - offer counselling and psychological support to patient and family
  - administer Rh prophylaxis if Rh-negative
  - give maternal steroids if preterm delivery is contemplated
  - after birth:
    - paediatric assessment and neurodevelopmental follow-up including MRI should be undertaken
    - post-mortem for the dead fetus should be discussed with parents
- At diagnosis:
  - check for signs of threatening miscarriage and severe preterm delivery
  - assess co-twin: fetal biometry, AFV, Doppler velocimetry and placental examination
- Dichorionic twins:
  - Doppler velocimetry (UA and MCA), fetal growth/biometry and AFV measurements every 2–4 weeks in the survivor
- Monochorionic twins:
  - continue fetal surveillance in surviving twin every one to two weeks: fetal growth/biometry assessment, AFV and Doppler velocimetry (UA and MCA +/-DV)
  - the MCA Doppler, recordings may suggest anemia, which, in turn, may predict the risk of brain damage; offer fetal blood transfusion if detected <35 weeks
  - consider offering an MRI at least three weeks after the time of presumed death to provide information about possible brain injury
- Timing and mode of delivery:
  - these should be discussed with the parents
  - recommendation in DC twins: deliver at 37^{+0}–37^{+6} weeks
  - recommendation in MC twins: deliver by 36^{+6} weeks
  - mode of delivery should be individualised, though tendency is for CS

(cont.)

TRAP Sequence

- Management options (empiric rather than evidence-based)
  - *conservative* when there is no evidence of hydramnios and/or hydrops
  - serial US surveillance: biometry including length as conventional measurements may be difficult in the acardiac twin, AFV, Doppler velocimetry
  - *intervention* when there is hydramnios and/or hydrops; aim is to stop the circulation in the acardiac twin
    - RFA from 16 weeks is the method most commonly reported.
    - Bipolar cord coagulation from 16 weeks seems to have more complications than RFA.
    - Limited data on intrafetal laser or MWA; the value of intrafetal laser before 16 weeks is being studied.

TTTS

- Management options:
  - expectant management
  - serial amnioreduction
  - septostomy
  - fetal laser ablation of vascular anastomoses – this is recommended as the first-line treatment by RCOG, SMFM, ISUOG and RANZCOG; centres offering this treatment should have operators with adequate training and experience
  - selective reduction.
- Perform MRI of the brains of the surviving fetuses four weeks after the procedure.
- Most authorities recommend elective delivery at 36^{+0}–37^{+0} weeks.
- Longer-term follow-up to two years of age is advocated.

TAPS

- Prenatal management options (dependent on gestational age, etiology of TAPS (spontaneous or post-operatively), accessibility of the placental vascular equator and severity of the condition)
  - elective delivery, especially if the condition presents late in pregnancy

(cont.)

- expectant management (especially if presenting in first or early second trimesters) comprising weekly fetal surveillance with UA and MCA Doppler velocimetry
- FBS and intrauterine/intraperitoneal fetal blood transfusions
- fetoscopic laser ablation of vascular anastomoses is the only curative treatment.
• Neonatal management
  - vigilance for anemia, polycythemia and/or thrombocytopenia
  - implement long-term neurodevelopmental surveillance.

Conjoined Twins

• Obtain careful ultrasonographic evaluation of anatomy; consider 3D US and/or MRI in addition.
• Provide interdisciplinary discussion of therapeutic options with the parents:
  - termination of pregnancy
  - continue with the pregnancy; prognosis depends on the amount and location of the shared tissue; whilst vaginal delivery may be possible if preterm labour occurs, most cases are delivered by CS; delivery should be in a tertiary centre with neonatal and paediatric surgical support.

3.2.5 Labour and Delivery

Planning Birth

Women should be given the opportunity to discuss mode and likely timing of birth from 24 weeks. Information should be tailored to the woman and her pregnancy and include discussion related to place of birth and potential need for transfer in case of PTB, timing and possible mode, analgesia, intrapartum fetal monitoring and management of the third stage [54].

Setting and Resources

Given the associated fetal and maternal risks of multiple pregnancy, delivery in an obstetric-led unit is routinely recommended to enable easy access to an obstetric operating theatre. Easy access to a specialist neonatal unit is vital. Since multiple pregnancies may require specialised and multidisciplinary support at the time of delivery, comprising immediate access to an experienced midwife, obstetrician, anaesthetist and neonatologist, is essential. Furthermore, if a preterm or operative delivery or fetal problems are anticipated, one neonatologist should be present per infant [54,94].

Timing of Birth

The mean duration of pregnancy of 138,660 twin gestations in the United States in 2008 was 35.3 weeks with a standard deviation of 3.6 weeks [319]. A study of 1,663 sets of twins from Germany published in 2020 found a median value of 35.0 weeks, with an interquartile range of 33–7 weeks [320]. It is difficult to establish to what extent these durations are shortened by intervention when complications arise because studying only spontaneous onset of labour excludes the large number of twin pregnancies with complications that would mean that they would have delivered early anyway, even without intervention. What is clear is that the peak risk of perinatal mortality for twin pregnancies occurs at an earlier gestational age than for singletons. Consequently, in twin pregnancies, early elective delivery is commonly recommended even when there are no obvious complications [321,322]. Chorionicity is a particularly important determinant of delivery timing. In the setting of DC twins, decisions relating to timing of delivery when complications arise are similar to those in singleton pregnancies. In the setting of MC pregnancies, decisions are complicated by the heightened risk of co-twin demise or adverse neurological sequelae in the event of single fetal death, owing to the shared circulation [257].

A 2016 systematic review and meta-analysis of 32 studies (29,685 DC and 5,486 MC twin pregnancies) examined the prospective weekly perinatal death risk following 37 weeks' gestation for uncomplicated DC twins and 36 weeks' gestation for uncomplicated MC twins, respectively. A delay in delivery to 38 weeks for DC twins led to an additional 8.8 perinatal deaths per 1,000 pregnancies (95% CI: 3.6–14.0/1,000, I^2 = 0%) compared with the previous week. A delay in delivery to 37 weeks for MC twins led to an additional 2.5 per 1,000 perinatal deaths, although that increase was not statistically significant [323]. A 2022 IPD meta-analysis aimed to elicit the effect of growth discordance or SGA on rates of stillbirth and NND. It demonstrated that growth discordance or SGA were associated with higher absolute risks of stillbirth and NND but, balancing these risks, there was no evidence to recommend a changing to the time of recommended delivery if growth disorders were present [227].

Amnionicity is also an important determinate in the timing of delivery for multiple gestations, with recommended delivery dates for MA twins being earlier than DA twins due to increased risks of single or double IUD within the third trimester due to a shared amnion. Currently there are no RCTs assessing the optimal timing of delivery for MCMA pregnancies. A 2019 meta-analysis of 25 studies (1,628 MCMA twins) demonstrated an overall incidence of fetal loss of approximately 6%, with rates greatest between 24 and 30 weeks' gestation [107]. Of these, 11 studies examined rates of IUD beyond 35 weeks, but the number of deaths were too few to draw significant conclusions. 37.8% (95% CI: 28.0–48.2%) of MCMA pregnancies were also delivered before the scheduled timing for delivery, due mainly to spontaneous PTB or abnormal cardiotocographic (CTG) findings [107].

Consequently, NICE, ACOG, ISUOG and RANZCOG recommend offering delivery [54,92,154,220]:

- at 37^{+0}–37^{+6} weeks for women with an uncomplicated DCDA twin pregnancy, because of the increased risk of fetal death from 38 weeks onwards.

The NICE guideline recommends offering delivery, following consideration of administration of corticosteroids [54]:

- at 36 weeks for women with an uncomplicated MCDA twin pregnancy because planned birth from 36^{+0} weeks does not appear to be associated with an increased risk of serious neonatal adverse outcome but that continuing the pregnancy beyond 36^{+6} weeks increases the risk of fetal death.
- between 32^{+0} and 33^{+6} weeks for women with an uncomplicated MCMA twin pregnancy.
- at 35 weeks for women with an uncomplicated TCTA or DCTA triplet pregnancy because continuing beyond 35^{+6} weeks increases the risk of fetal death.

Conduct of Labour

Multiple pregnancies have a greater intrapartum blood loss than singletons and an increased rate of PPH, and thus intravenous access, full blood count, and serum group and save should be obtained early in labour, with the consideration of prophylactic uterotonics following delivery [5,94]. Continuous fetal monitoring should occur once there are regular contractions. Care must be exercised to ensure that two distinct heart rate tracings are being obtained. Until the membranes of the first twin have ruptured, this will be via external transducers, and thus it is important to use a twin monitor to allow simultaneous recording with the option of separating the heart rates by adding 20 beats/min to one. Ideally, after membrane rupture, the first twin should be monitored by a fetal scalp electrode (unless contraindicated). It is still important to continually check at each CTG assessment that two distinct fetal heart rate (FHR) traces are being obtained. Fetal scalp stimulation should not be used in twin pregnancy to 'gain reassurance' from a pathological classification of the CTG. Twin pregnancy should be considered a fetal clinical risk factor when performing CTG classification. This should lower the threshold for identification of fetal concerns in a way similar to that which should occur in the presence of meconium [54]. With suspected fetal compromise of the leading twin at ≥34 weeks' gestation, scalp FBS is appropriate, and the findings should be interpreted as in singleton pregnancy [54]. However, a frank discussion about the ultimate likelihood of recourse to caesarean section is important. According to NICE, women with uncomplicated pregnancies giving birth after 32 weeks should be advised that more than one-third of women that plan a vaginal birth will go on to have a caesarean and that a small number will need an emergency caesarean for the second twin after vaginal birth of the first [54].

Epidural anaesthesia should be discussed not only in the context of pain relief for labour but also in the event that interventions are required for delivery, in particular of the second twin (e.g., operative delivery or internal podalic version (IPV)). Augmentation by using oxytocin may be used.

Mode of Delivery

Before delivery, the woman should understand the potential complications, including spontaneous change in fetal presentation and the risk of either instrumental vaginal delivery and/or emergency caesarean section. Fetal presentation at the time of labour and delivery may not correspond to what was seen at the last antenatal assessment, which is the case in nearly one-third of pregnancies last scanned at 32–6 weeks [79]. Fetal lie must be determined on admission with US in all cases, and potentially intrapartum. Successful delivery management is reliant upon preparation and well-coordinated multidisciplinary care.

The three clinically relevant combinations of fetal presentations for twin gestations are:

- cephalic–cephalic
- cephalic–non-cephalic
- both non-cephalic

There needs to be consideration of other risk factors when planning mode of delivery such as previous caesarean section and PTB. Monoamniotic and higher-order multiples also require special consideration.

Cephalic–Cephalic Presentation

This is the most common presentation in twins, representing 40% at delivery. Malpresentation of one or both twins occurs in 60%: vertex–non-vertex in 35–40% and non-vertex–non-vertex or vertex in 20% [324]. Recommendations regarding the optimal mode of delivery are primarily guided by the presentation of the first twin (twin A). Birthweight difference in relation to the presenting twin, gestational age, senior clinician skill and experience, and patient preference are other key determinants [325]. The consensus is that if both twins are in cephalic presentation, a vaginal delivery can be offered even in the setting of LBW (<1,500 g) [28], unless a specific contraindication to vaginal birth exists [29]. The recommendation of NICE is that vaginal birth and planned caesarean section are both safe choices for DC and MC pregnancies, if the first twin is cephalic, the pregnancy has been uncomplicated and passed 32 weeks and there is no significant size discordance [54].

Non-cephalic Twin A

In the case of a non-cephalic-presenting twin A, RCOG, NICE and RANZCOG currently recommend an elective caesarean section [54,220,326]. However, it is recognised that there are limitations to the volume of available high-quality evidence to underpin this recommendation. The evidence in singletons is from the Term Breech Trial, which investigated delivery for singleton breech cases. It concluded that planned caesarean section is associated with substantially improved neonatal outcomes [327]. This trial was included in a 2015 Cochrane review that concluded that whilst perinatal death or NND (excluding fatal anomalies) was reduced with planned caesarean section (RR: 0.29, 95% CI: 0.10–0.86, three studies, 2,388 women), there was a reported higher risk of short-term maternal morbidity following a policy of planned caesarean (RR: 1.29, 95% CI: 1.03–1.61, three studies, 2,396 women, low-quality evidence) [328]. These results can be extrapolated to the first twin only. A 2003 systematic review assessed caesarean delivery in twins compared to vaginal birth and included three cohort studies and a single RCT and demonstrated that a low Apgar score at 5 min was less frequent in those delivered by planned caesarean section (OR: 0.47, 95% CI: 0.26–0.88) but these twins spent significantly longer in hospital [329]. Conversely, a 2012 systematic review of 16 observational studies of non-cephalic twin A presentation did not demonstrate a benefit of caesarean section in non-cephalic-presenting twins but highlighted the small sample sizes of the included studies [330]. A 2020 national prospective population-based study of 1,467 twin deliveries did not find a significant difference in neonatal mortality and morbidity of vaginal breech delivery of the first twin compared to caesarean section (adjusted RR: 0.71, 95% CI: 0.27–1.86) [331]. More robust, high-quality evidence is required to make firm decisions on mode of delivery for non-cephalic twin A presentations, taking into account gestation, chorionicity and other risk factors. However, at the time of writing, there is general consensus that if the first twin is a non-cephalic presentation, then caesarean section should be offered.

Limited research is available on the applicability of external cephalic version (ECV) for non-vertex-presenting twins. A recent systematic review of two case reports and a small case series of 22 patients demonstrated a 57% success rate in ECV for mispositioned presenting twins, with 85% of successful interventions proceeding to an uncomplicated vaginal delivery [332]. Further research is required in this area to universally recommend this procedure, which is technically challenging.

Cephalic Twin A plus Non-cephalic Twin B

In the setting of a non-vertex twin B, RCOG recommends vaginal delivery by breech extraction provided the infant weighs >1,500 g and all other criteria for vaginal breech delivery are met [333]. A 2011 systematic review and meta-analysis of 18 studies (39,571 twin pairs) confirmed lower neonatal morbidity (3.0 vs 4.6%, OR: 0.53, 95% CI: 0.39–0.70, p <0.001) and mortality for the first compared to the second twin (0.3 vs 0.6%, OR: 0.55, 95% CI: 0.38–0.81, p = 0.02), regardless of mode of delivery [334]. There was no difference in morbidity between twins in cephalic and non-cephalic presentations or for planned method of delivery. A significant difference in neonatal morbidity was identified when the second twin had to be delivered by emergency caesarean section after vaginal delivery of the first. In this instance, morbidity was higher for the second twin compared to vaginal birth or planned caesarean section (19.8 vs 9.5 vs 9.8%; p <0.0001) [334].

In 2013, a multicentre prospective RCT, the Twin Birth Study, published its results, which have been used to derive a lot of the recommendations made in the RCOG twin birth guidance [335]. This included deliveries between 32 and 38^{+6} weeks' gestation, with a DA twin pregnancy (25% MC) and the first twin in the cephalic presentation. Participants were randomised to either planned caesarean section or planned vaginal birth. Primary outcome was a composite of fetal or NND or serious neonatal morbidity. In the planned CS group, 89.9% had CS for both babies, 9.3% delivered both twins vaginally, and in 0.8% (n = 11) of cases, the second twin was delivered via CS following the vaginal birth of the first twin. In the planned vaginal birth group, both twins were born vaginally in 56.2% of cases, in 39.6% of cases both were born by CS and in 4.2% the second twin was delivered via CS after the vaginal birth of the first. There was no significant difference in the mortality and overall morbidity of mothers and children in the two groups, at 7.3 versus 8.5% (OR: 0.86, 95% CI: 0.65–1.13, p = 0.29) and 2.2 versus 1.9% (OR: 1.16, 95% CI: 0.77–1.74, p = 0.45). Regardless of the delivery method, the overall risk of morbidity was significantly higher for the second twin than for the first (OR: 1.9, 95% CI: 1.34–2.69, p <0.001). It can be concluded that under these conditions, for both DC and MC pregnancies there are no benefits of planned CS compared to planned vaginal birth for twins between 32 and 38 weeks' gestation when the first twin is cephalic [335]. Longer-term follow-up of the babies in the trial has demonstrated no benefit at two years of age with a policy of planned caesarean delivery [336]. It should be noted that the obstetricians involved in this study were highly skilled in the management of vaginal birth of both twins, as there were relatively few cases of combined vaginal and caesarean births (4.2%). As such, all obstetricians should take note of the recommendations by RCOG and within the literature, whilst focusing on maintaining their skillset to manage twin deliveries in their respective labour ward units [312].

A 2014 WHO global survey on outcomes for 1,424 twin pregnancies demonstrated 25.9% of this cohort had a non-vertex second twin presentation. Of this patient subgroup, the rate of caesarean section was significantly greater than in second twin vertex presentation (6.2 vs 0.9%, p <0.001) [337]. However, although rates of low Apgar score (<7) at 5 min were reported to be significantly greater (16.0 vs 11.4%, AOR: 1.42, 95% CI: 1.01–2.00) in non-vertex-presenting second twins, the rates of stillbirth, NND and admission to NICU were not different [337]. Similar results have been reported by observational studies. These same studies showed conflicting results as to whether a non-cephalic presentation of the second twin was a risk factor for caesarean section for that twin [338,339]. Thus, at present, the evidence suggest that vaginal delivery of the non-cephalic (breech) second twin presentation when the presenting twin is cephalic is as safe as vaginal delivery of twins in the vertex–vertex presentation.

Previous Caesarean Section

Women with twin pregnancies who have had a previous cesarean section are less likely to attempt a vaginal birth after cesarean section (VBAC) but they are no more likely to fail a VBAC trial compared to women with singleton gestations [340]. Studies have reported no difference in perinatal outcomes for twins delivered vaginally or by elective caesarean section in twin pregnancies following previous caesarean section [341,342,343]. A retrospective multicentre study of 236 twin trials of labour after caesarean section reported in 2022 found no significant difference in the rates of uterine rupture between vertex–vertex and vertex–non-vertex presentations, including no difference in maternal morbidity, neonatal morbidity or mortality [342]. This contrasts with a systematic review published in 2021 of four retrospective studies that reported that the rate of uterine rupture was significantly higher in the twins undergoing vaginal birth after prior caesarean section rather than planned caesarean (OR: 9.43, 95% CI: 3.54–25.17), although absolute rates of uterine rupture were very low regardless of mode of delivery (0.87 vs 0.09%, respectively) [343].

Caesarean Section

Compared with vaginal birth, it is known that infants born by caesarean are at greater risk of respiratory distress syndrome (RDS), transient tachypnoea of the newborn (TTN) and admission to NICU, with risks decreasing as gestational age increases [344,345]. A 2016 study reported that caesarean delivery significantly increased the frequency of RDS in both twins compared with vaginal birth, but only at gestational ages <30 weeks [346]. Accordingly, the advisability of prophylactic corticosteroids should take into account primarily gestational age, fetal size and associated comorbidities and follow the same guidance as for singleton pregnancies. The 2022 RCOG guidelines state

> For women undergoing planned caesarean birth between 37^{+0} and 38^{+6} weeks an informed discussion should take place with the woman about the potential risks and benefits of a course of antenatal corticosteroids. Although antenatal corticosteroids may reduce admission to the neonatal unit for respiratory morbidity, it is uncertain if there is any reduction in RDS, transient tachypnoea of the newborn or neonatal unit admission overall and antenatal corticosteroids may result in harm to the neonate which includes hypoglycaemia and potential developmental delay [347].

Evidence suggests that mothers and infants spend significantly longer in hospital if delivered by caesarean section, albeit maternal stay may significantly bias these figures [348].

In summary, there is no evidence to suggest that caesarean section confers an improvement in maternal or fetal morbidity or mortality, unless twin A is non-vertex. In the context of acute intrapartum care, such as cord prolapse, placental abruption, fetal compromise or malpresentation of the second twin, combined delivery with secondary emergency caesarean section for the second twin may be necessary. Women who elect to have vaginal birth should thus be aware of the risk of combined delivery in the setting of multiple pregnancy [54].

Preterm or LBW Twin Birth

It should be noted that the majority of evidence recommended so far relates to pregnancies >32 weeks' gestation and fetal weight >1,500 g. The evidence for mode of delivery in preterm twin pregnancies is mainly encompassed by retrospective studies analysing outcomes of neonatal morbidity and mortality. There is available evidence to promote vaginal birth of both twins, some reporting equivocal outcomes between modes of delivery and some supporting caesarean section with an increase in neonatal mortality if twin weights are <1,500 g [349,350,351].

In the context of extremely preterm twin gestations, there is a paucity of data with regards to a recommended mode of delivery. A 2017 systematic review of extremely preterm twins (24^{+0}–27^{+6}) demonstrated no significant difference between composite outcomes of NND and severe brain injury for cephalic–non-cephalic twins delivering either vaginally or by caesarean section (95% CI: 0.05–13.43, two studies, $I^2 = 56\%$) [352]. A 2020 retrospective study of 390 twin gestations drew similar conclusions [353]. However, Tucker Edmonds et al. provided evidence to support that overall survival was greater for caesarean-born neonates at previable gestations; both 23 and 24 weeks' gestations (AOR: 3.98, 95% CI: 2.24–7.06, AOR: 2.91, 95% CI: 1.76–4.81, respectively) [354]. There is an urgent need for research in this area, and at present, mode of delivery will need to be individualised according to gestation, BW, fetal condition and indication for delivery, after appropriate counselling of parents.

MA Twins and Higher-Order Multiples

Caesarean section is the recommended mode of birth for MCMA twins due to the risk of cord entanglement and inter-twin locking [54,233]. For higher-order multiples, caesarean is also the recommended mode of birth [54].

Delivery Procedures

Cephalic–Cephalic Presentation: Vaginal Delivery

Late second-stage management of delivery for twin A should be as for singleton vaginal birth. Following delivery, delayed cord clamping (DCC) may be permitted based on the presumed extrapolation of benefits for term singletons. However, the cord should be clamped immediately if contraindications to DCC are known, such as the need to immediately resuscitate neonate or mother, fetal hydrops or utero-placental haemorrhage [355]. The literature on the effects of DCC in term twin births is sparse, in part because studies have not exclusively analysed twin deliveries or analysed the twin data subgroup within a larger cohort. Delayed cord clamping in preterm twins has produced some possible evidence of benefit. A recent observational study of 624 twins demonstrated DCC in preterm infants was associated with a reduced need for delivery room intubation (AOR: 0.53, 95% CI: 0.42–0.68), mechanical ventilation (AOR: 0.51, 95% CI: 0.39–0.67) and NICU length of stay (adjusted coefficient –4.17, 95% CI: 8.15 to –0.19) [356]. However, results should be interpreted cautiously, as babies eligible for DCC at birth are likely to be from more stable patients who would otherwise have less of a risk of adverse outcomes irrespective of DCC or not. A recent small cohort study of 58 patients did not show any difference in outcomes with DCC compared to immediate [357]. A 2019 RCT demonstrated minimal benefit for DCC compared to immediate with regards to superior vena cava flow, admission haematocrit and levels at eight weeks; however, incidence of maternal PPH was higher in the DCC group (4.3% in ICC vs 25% in DCC, p = 0.04) [358]. For uncomplicated MC twins, delayed umbilical cord clamping should not be practiced due to an increased risk of acute feto-fetal haemorrhage due to the placental vascular anastomoses.

Vaginal delivery of the second twin remains a challenge in obstetric practice. Uterine inertia, abnormal lie or a high presenting part of the second twin may occur following delivery of the first twin. Accurate determination and stabilisation of the lie of the second twin must be obtained immediately by an experienced obstetrician, and US examination may be required when the lie is not readily ascertainable by abdominal palpation or vaginal examination. Only once fetal lie is firmly established, and the presenting part is confirmed to not be high, is it safe to perform artificial rupture of membranes. A scalp electrode may be applied at this time if in vertex position, to maintain accurate fetal monitoring, given the increased risk of intrapartum asphyxia.

Oxytocin infusion is valuable in the setting of reduced contractility or uterine inertia, or when there is perceived to be insufficient maternal effort to achieve timely delivery of twin B, but should only be given after it has been determined that twin B is in a position suitable for delivery. Giving oxytocin before this risks losing the opportunity for IPV due to a reduction in intrauterine volume as it contracts the uterus, preventing the baby being turned. For some cephalic–cephalic births, a vertex delivery will not occur for the second twin because of a change in presentation after delivery of the first twin, fetal compromise, cord prolapse or failure of engagement. Thus, between 0.8 and 3.9% will require breech extraction and up to 10% will require emergency caesarean section [335,359,360].

Cephalic–Non-cephalic Delivery of Second Twin

In the setting of a transverse or oblique twin B, fetal lie requires correction by an experienced obstetrician. One option is ECV (Figure 7), which aims to

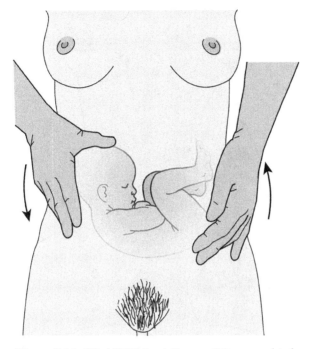

Figure 7 Modified ECV for delivery of the second twin

manipulate the fetal head over the pelvic inlet to a vertex position. However, in the context of vaginal breech with intact membranes, IPV followed by breech extraction (Figure 8) appears to be associated with a significantly lower incidence of fetal compromise and abdominal delivery with comparable neonatal outcome [361]. The Twin Birth Study demonstrated a 95% success rate in patients delivered by breech extraction, compared with 42% by ECV, confirming that breech extraction is the optimal procedure for the non-vertex second twin [335]. In both cases, the membranes should remain intact as this aids manoeuvres and reduces the risk of cord prolapse [335]. Internal podalic version comprises a series of manoeuvres performed prior to breech extraction and may also be used to expedite delivery in the case of profound bradycardia (Figure 8). Adequate analgesia is however an essential prerequisite, as is informed verbal consent by the woman.

Throughout delivery, continuous FHR monitoring should be maintained. The bladder is first emptied and the woman positioned in the lithotomy position. The responsible obstetrician should then locate the fetal foot by internal palpation. Once it has been identified, the membranes may be artificially ruptured, and one or (preferably) both feet are held and guided down to the vagina. Assisted breech delivery is then performed to achieve safe delivery of the second twin.

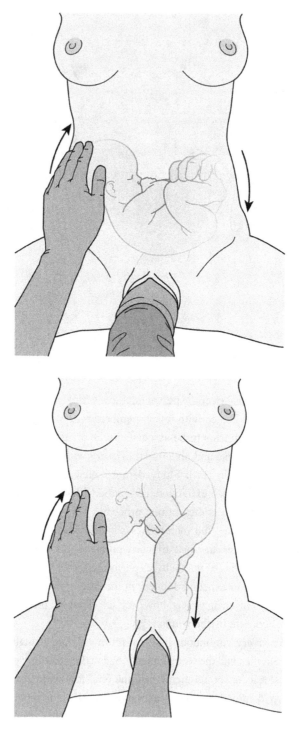

Figure 8 Internal podalic version for delivery of the second twin

Potential complications of IPV include:

- fetal anoxia
- failed delivery
- trauma (e.g., hip dislocation)
- inadvertent delivery of a hand/shoulder
- placental abruption
- cord prolapse
- endometritis
- maternal trauma – inversion, rupture

There is increasing evidence to suggest a rapid decline in the use of breech extraction, with a concomitant decrease in IPV, despite its high success rate [362]. There is thus an urgent need to ensure that obstetricians are trained and remain competent and confident in these manoeuvres.

Time Interval between Delivery of Twins

A retrospective study performed by Stein et al. assessed the correlation between the twin-to-twin delivery interval and umbilical blood gas of the second twin in 4,110 twin deliveries ≥34 weeks following vaginal delivery of the first twin. The mean twin-to-twin delivery time interval was 13.5 min (SD: 17.1 min). However, the majority of the second twins, 3,115 (75.8%) were born within 15 min after delivery of the first twin (the time distribution was not Gaussian). Some 674 (16.4%) second twins were born within 16–30 min, 178 (4.3%) within 31–45 min, 71 (1.7%) within 46–60 min and 72 (1.8%) after >60 min. A significant negative correlation between delivery interval and cord blood gas was demonstrated. With a delivery interval of 0–15 min, umbilical arterial pH of twin B was <7.10 (OR: 1). with a delivery interval of 16–30 min, the rate of pH at <7.1 of the second twin increased (OR: 3.5, 95% CI: 2–6.3), with a delivery interval of 31–45 min (OR: 5.2, 95% CI: 2.4–11.5), with a delivery interval of 46–60 min (OR: 6.7, 95% CI: 2.5–17.7) and with a delivery interval of >60 min (OR: 9.3, 95% CI: 3.6–23.8) [363]. A study of 527 twin deliveries also demonstrated a significant negative association between UA pH and interval twin delivery (0–30 min pH 7.23 and >30 min pH 7.20, p <0.0001) [364]. Some authors have recommended that an inter-twin delivery interval of less than 30 min should be achieved to reduce the risk of compromise and acidosis in the second twin [364,365]. However, studies have shown no increased risk in perinatal morbidity or mortality with increasing inter-twin delivery interval if continuous fetal monitoring is used [364,366,367].

In view of the conflicting evidence, it would seem sensible that no limit is put on the time interval but that the aim of management for the second twin is to ensure that there is adequate fetal monitoring with CTG (external or internal) and that the delivery is actively managed by a senior obstetrician. This involves not only assessing fetal wellbeing, considering current CTG, CTG during first stage and risk factors for fetal compromise, but also maternal condition and ensuring that there are adequate contractions. When delivery needs to be expedited because of concerns regarding fetal condition, this may be achieved by operative vacuum, forceps or breech extraction.

Twin Entrapment

If twin A presents breech, and twin B is cephalic presentation, there is a risk of twin entrapment in the setting of vaginal delivery. This occurs when the head of the second twin enters the pelvis prior to the head of the presenting twin, thus obstructing labour progression. This is an obstetric emergency, associated with fetal death of the first twin and perinatal asphyxia for both [102]. Attempts to release the locked twins by internal manual manoeuvres that push the first twin back into the pelvis may be performed to enable the cephalic second twin to deliver first. However, if this is unsuccessful, an emergency caesarean section is indicated.

Third Stage of Labour

All women with twin or triplet pregnancy should be offered active management of the third stage, as it is associated with a lower risk of PPH and/or blood transfusion [54]. Additional uterotonics for the active management of the third stage should be considered if additional risk factors are present (other than just multiple gestation) for PPH [54].

SUMMARY OF MANAGEMENT OPTIONS

Labour and Delivery
Planning Birth, Setting and Resources

- Parents should have a prenatal discussion of the management/conduct of labour and delivery.
- Advise delivery in an obstetric unit.
- An experienced obstetrician and anaesthetist to be available for labour and delivery; a neonatal paediatrician and neonatal team to be available for delivery, with one paediatrician present per infant if a preterm or operative delivery or fetal problems are anticipated.

(cont.)

Timing of Birth

The most recent update of the NICE guideline recommends offering planned birth:

- at 37^{+0}–37^{+6} weeks for an uncomplicated DCDA twin pregnancy.
- after considering administration of corticosteroids:
  - at 36 weeks for an uncomplicated MCDA twin pregnancy
  - at 32^{+0}–33^{+6} weeks for an uncomplicated MCMA twin pregnancy.
- at 35 weeks for an uncomplicated TCTA or DCTA triplet pregnancy.

Conduct of Labour and Delivery

- Obtain intravenous access at onset of labour; take blood for full blood count and serum for blood group and saving it if needed for a blood transfusion.
- Maintain continuous fetal monitoring of both twins throughout labour, ensuring distinction of the two heart rates.
- Be aware that the second twin is at highest risk of adverse outcome whether delivered vaginally or by CS.
- Epidural analgesia is recommended.
- Consider synthetic oxytocin infusion for uterine inertia, especially after the first twin is delivered (should not be given until a favourable position of twin B is established).

Mode of Delivery

- Choice is influenced by presentation, BW difference, gestational age and patient preferences.
- Caesarean section is recommended for MCMA and higher-order multiples.
- The following recommendations relate to twin pregnancies at 32^{+0} weeks or more.
- **Cephalic twin A–cephalic twin B**
  - Consensus is that a vaginal delivery should be advised in the absence of a contraindication to vaginal birth.
  - Establish fetal lie of twin B after twin A delivered, ideally with US.
  - Perform amniotomy provided the presenting part is not high and a longitudinal lie is confirmed; continue FHR monitoring.

(cont.)

- **Non-cephalic twin A**
  - RCOG/NICE recommend elective CS.
- **Cephalic twin A–non-cephalic twin B**
  - ACOG and RCOG recommend vaginal birth for twin A and breech extraction/vaginal delivery for twin B.
  - Establish fetal lie of twin B after twin A delivered, ideally with US.
  - An experienced obstetrician to perform IPV followed by breech extraction; this has a higher success rate than ECV.
  - With IPV or ECV, membranes should ideally remain intact until the manoeuvre is completed.
  - Continuous FHR monitoring throughout.
  - Epidural 'top-up' is advisable before an assisted delivery.
- There is no evidence to justify a set inter-twin birth interval; the priority is to ensure both have FHR monitoring.
- Twin entrapment occurs generally with breech twin A and vertex twin B presentation: management options are a) manually pushing the first twin back into the uterus and deliver the second twin first or, b) an emergency CS.

Preterm or LBW Twin Birth

- In preterm labour <32 weeks or where EFW of the fetus is <1,500 g, there is conflicting opinion about the optimal mode of delivery and little evidence to guide decision-making, thus, mode of delivery should be individualised depending on gestation, BWs, conditions of the fetuses and indication/reason for delivery, and a detailed discussion with the parents.

Third Stage of Labour

- Active management is advocated; extra uterotonics may be required.

3.2.6 Postnatal

General

Although the principles of postnatal care do not differ from those that apply to singleton births, women with multiple pregnancies may require additional support. The postnatal hospital care of women with multiple births may in the first instance be prolonged, and additional community support may also be required postnatally. All mothers should receive adequate encouragement and support to successfully establish breastfeeding, and in the context of multiple birth, this may demand increased healthcare team input. Women should also receive contraceptive advice early in the postnatal period to avoid an unintended pregnancy, and ideally these conversations should begin antenatally.

A heightened awareness for postnatal depression may be justified. Research in this area is limited, however, a 2015 systematic review has demonstrated an increased occurrence in mothers of multiple gestations compared to singletons [368]. Recognised risk factors for postnatal depression, such as pre-eclampsia, hyperemesis, emergency caesarean or instrumental delivery, premature delivery and excessive bleeding intrapartum, are higher for this group [367,368]. Offspring are also more likely to require neonatal unit admission in the immediate postpartum period. Socioeconomic deprivation indicators such as unemployment, low income and low education have been cited as risk factors in mental health disorders [368,369]. The added financial implications associated with multiple birth are thus likely to be relevant.

A good domestic relationship and positive social support are considered protective factors against postnatal depression and may be particularly valuable in this context [368,369]. Maintaining or establishing contact with the local multiple birth support groups during the puerperium may also be important.

SUMMARY OF MANAGEMENT OPTIONS

Postnatal

- Provide extra support while in hospital to assist with infant care.
- Encourage breastfeeding.
- Offer longer inpatient stay.
- Arrange support at home.
- Increased vigilance for maternal postnatal mental health problems.
- Provide adequate contraceptive advice.

4 Higher-Order Multiples Summary

Triplet and higher-order multiple pregnancies are particularly high-risk groups and warrant separate consideration. Internationally, an overall decline in triplet pregnancies is observed, which likely reflects statutory regulation of AR practice [1]. Multifetal pregnancies are associated with a higher risk of maternal, perinatal and long-term complications when compared to singletons or twins [219]. Although modern neonatal care has improved survival rates of preterm as well as LBW triplets, with 2014 rates showing comparable perinatal mortality for twins and triplets, significant complications still exist [370]. Because of these issues and the additional challenges in fetal surveillance, early referral to a tertiary centre with a specialist fetal medicine service from initial diagnosis is required [312]. The subject of MFPR is relevant in this setting, and even in triplet pregnancies, reduced rates of pregnancy loss, antenatal complications, PTB, LBW and NND have been reported with reduction [240].

To reflect the increased risks associated with triplet pregnancies, closer maternal and fetal monitoring is recommended [54]. For those pregnancies with a shared chorion, increased fetal growth surveillance is recommended and may commence from 16 weeks' gestation at two-weekly intervals. Recommendations vary for monitoring in TCTA pregnancies, with some suggesting that they may requires less intensive growth surveillance [371]. Scans every 14 days from 20 weeks are recommended by NICE [146]. Before screening is performed, women should receive clear counselling regarding the greater likelihood of Down syndrome. In terms of screening, only NT and maternal age are utilised in this setting, and thus the accuracy of testing is also lower.

A particularly important complication in higher-order multiples is PTB, especially given its associations with perinatal mortality and long-term child morbidity [73]. Concerning mode of delivery, the potential difficulties with electronic fetal monitoring, unrecognised hypoxemia (especially given the high incidence of FGR) and birth trauma from manipulative delivery of non-cephalic -presenting fetuses mean that caesarean section is generally advocated in triplet and higher-order multiple pregnancies [54].

Summary of Management Options

Higher-Order Multiples

- All cases require early referral to a tertiary centre with a specialist fetal medicine service.
- Only NT and maternal age can be used for screening for aneuploidy.
- If invasive prenatal diagnosis is required, amniocentesis is the preferred option.
- Growth surveillance
  a) commence at 16 weeks and at two-weekly intervals for triplets with a shared chorion
  b) commence at 20 weeks and at four-weekly intervals for TCTA pregnancies.

(cont.)
- MFPR (see Section 3.2.4) should be discussed as higher-order multiple pregnancies are associated with reduced rates of pregnancy loss, antenatal complications, PTB, LBW and NND.
- Most advocate elective caesarean section for delivery of triplet and higher-order births.

Abbreviations

AA	arterio-arterial
AC	abdominal circumference
ACOG	American College of Obstetricians and Gynecologists
AFV	amniotic fluid volume
AOR	adjusted odds ratio
AR	assisted reproduction
AV	arterio-venous
β-hCG	β-human chorionic gonadotropin
BMI	body mass index
BW	birthweight
cffDNA	cell-free fetal DNA
CI	confidence interval
CL	cervical length
CRL	crown rump length
CTG	cardiotocographic
CVS	chorionic villus sampling
DA	diamniotic
DC	dichorionic
DCC	delayed cord clamping
DCTA	dichorionic triamniotic
DET	double embryo transfer
DNA	deoxyribonucleic acid
DV	ductus venosus
DVP	deepest vertical pocket
DZ	dizygotic
ECV	external cephalic version
EFW	estimated fetal weight
EPPPIC	Evaluating Progestogens for Preventing Preterm Birth International Collaborative

eSET	elective single embryo transfer
ESPRIT	Evaluation of Sonographic Predictors of Restricted Growth in Twins
FBS	fetal blood sampling
fFN	fetal fibronectin
FGR	fetal growth restriction
FIGO	The International Federation of Gynecology and Obstetrics
FLA	fetoscopic laser ablation
FMF	Fetal Medicine Foundation
fMRI	fetal magnetic resonance imaging
Hb	hemaglobin
HC	head circumference
HFEA	Human Fertilisation and Embryology Authority
ICP	intrahepatic cholestasis of pregnancy
ICSI	intracytoplasmic sperm injection
IM	intramuscular
IPD	individual patient data
IPV	internal podalic version
ISPD	International Society for Prenatal Diagnosis
ISUOG	International Society of Ultrasound in Obstetrics and Gynecology
IUD	intrauterine death
IUT	intrauterine transfusion
IVF	in vitro fertilisation
LBW	low birthweight
MA	monoamniotic
MBRRACE	Mothers and Babies: Reducing Risk through Audits and Confidential Enquiries
MC	monochorionic
MCA	middle cerebral artery
MCDA	monochorionic diamniotic
MCMA	monochorionic monoamniotic
MCTA	monochorionic triamniotic
MFPR	multifetal pregnancy reduction
MPJ	membrane-placental junction
MWA	microwave ablation
MZ	monozygotic
NICE	National Institute for Health and Care Excellence
NICU	neonatal intensive care unit
NIHCD	National Institute of Child Health and Human Development

NIPT	non-invasive prenatal testing
NND	neonatal death
NSC	National Screening Committee
NT	nuchal translucency
ONS	Office for National Statistics
OR	odds ratio
PAPP-A	pregnancy-associated plasma protein A
PI	pulsatility index
PPH	postpartum haemorrhage
PPROM	preterm prelabour rupture of membranes
PSV	peak systolic velocity
PTB	preterm birth
PZ	polyzygotic
RANZCOG	Royal Australian and New Zealand College of Obstetricians and Gynaecologists
RCOG	Royal College of Obstetricians and Gynaecologists
RCT	randomised controlled trial
RDS	respiratory distress syndrome
RFA	radiofrequency ablation
RR	relative risk
SET	single embryo transfer
sFGR	selective fetal growth restriction
SGA	small for gestational age
sIUFD	single intrauterine fetal demise
SMFM	Society for Maternal–Fetal Medicine
SOGC	Society Obstetricians and Gynecologists of Canada
SR	selective reduction
STORK	Southwest Thames Obstetric Research Collaborative
TAPS	twin anemia–polycythemia sequence
TCTA	trichorionic triamniotic
TOP	termination of pregnancy
TRAP	twin reversed arterial perfusion
TTN	transient tachypnoea of the newborn
TTTS	twin-to-twin transfusion syndrome
UA	umbilical artery
US	ultrasound
VTS	vanishing twin syndrome
VV	veno-venous
WHO	World Health Organisation

Further Reading

Farmer, N, Hillier, M, Kilby, MD, Hodgetts-Morton, V, Morris, RK. Outcomes in intervention and management of multiple pregnancies trials: a systematic review. Eur J Obstet Gynecol Reprod Biol. 2021; 261: 178–92.

Khalil, A, Rodgers, M, Baschat, A, et al. ISUOG practice guidelines: role of ultrasound in twin pregnancy. Ultrasound Obstet Gynecol. 2016; 47: 247–63.

Mackie, FL, Rigby, A, Morris, RK, Kilby, MD. Prognosis of the co-twin following spontaneous single intrauterine fetal death in twin pregnancies: a systematic review and meta-analysis. BJOG. 2019; 126: 569–78.

di Mascio, D, Acharya, G, Khalil, A, et al. Birthweight discordance and neonatal morbidity in twin pregnancies: a systematic review and meta-analysis. Acta Obstet Gynecol Scand. 2019; 98: 1245–57.

d'Antonio, F, Odibo, A, Berghella, V, et al. Perinatal mortality, timing of delivery and prenatal management of monoamniotic twin pregnancy: systematic review and meta-analysis. Ultrasound Obstet Gynecol. 2019; 53: 166–74.

Khalil, A, Beune, I, Hecher, K, et al. Consensus definition and essential reporting parameters of selective fetal growth restriction in twin pregnancy: a Delphi procedure. Ultrasound Obstet Gynecol. 2019; 53: 47–54.

Royal College of Obstetricians and Gynaecologists (RCOG). Management of Monochorionic Twin Pregnancy, 2nd edn. Green-top Guideline No. 51. London: RCOG, 2016. www.rcog.org.uk/en/guidelines-research-services/guidelines/gtg51/ (accessed 13 September 2024).

Khalil, A, Gordijn, S, Ganzevoort, W, et al. Consensus diagnostic criteria and monitoring of twin anemia–polycythemia sequence: Delphi procedure. Ultrasound Obstet Gynecol. 2020; 56: 388–94.

National Institute for Health and Care Excellence (NICE). Twin and Triplet Pregnancy. NICE Guideline NG137. London: NICE, 2024. www.nice.org.uk/guidance/ng137 (accessed 22nd October 2024).

di Mascio, D, Khalil, A, Rizzo, G, et al. Risk of fetal loss following amniocentesis or chorionic villus sampling in twin pregnancy: systematic review and meta-analysis. Ultrasound Obstet Gynecol. 2020; 56: 647–55.

Multifetal gestations: twin, triplet, and higher-order multifetal pregnancies: ACOG practice bulletin, number 231. Obstet Gynecol. 2021; 137: e145–62.

Nicholas, L, Fischbein, R, Ernst-Milner, S, Wani, R. Review of international clinical guidelines related to prenatal screening during monochorionic pregnancies. J Clin Med. 2021; 10: 1128.

Townsend, R, d'Antonio, F, Sileo, FG, et al. Perinatal outcome of monochorionic twin pregnancy complicated by selective fetal growth restriction according to management: systematic review and meta-analysis. Ultrasound Obstet Gynecol. 2019; 53: 36–46.

Marleen, S, Dias, C, Nandasena, R, et al. Association between chorionicity and preterm birth in twin pregnancies: a systematic review involving 29 864 twin pregnancies. BJOG. 2021; 128: 788–96.

EPPPIC Group. Evaluating Progestogens for Preventing Preterm birth International Collaborative (EPPPIC): meta-analysis of individual participant data from randomised controlled trials. Lancet. 2021; 397: 1183–94.

Romero, R, Conde-Agudelo, A, Rehal, A, et al. Vaginal progesterone for the prevention of preterm birth and adverse perinatal outcomes in twin gestations with a short cervix: an updated individual patient data meta-analysis. Ultrasound Obstet Gynecol. 2022; 59: 263–6.

Li, C, Shen, J, Hua, K. Cerclage for women with twin pregnancies: a systematic review and meta-analysis. Am J Obstet Gynecol. 2019; 220: 543–55.

Donepudi, R, Hessami, K, Nassr, AA, et al. Selective reduction in complicated monochorionic pregnancies: a systematic review and meta-analysis of different techniques. Am J Obstet Gynecol. 2022; 226: 646–55.

di Mascio, D, Khalil, A, d'Amico, A, et al. Outcome of twin–twin transfusion syndrome according to Quintero stage of disease: systematic review and meta-analysis. Ultrasound Obstet Gynecol. 2020; 56: 811–20.

Murgano, D, Khalil, A, Prefumo, F, et al. Outcome of twin-to-twin transfusion syndrome in monochorionic monoamniotic twin pregnancy: systematic review and meta-analysis. Ultrasound Obstet Gynecol. 2020; 55: 310–17.

References

1 Office for National Statistics. Birth Characteristics in England and Wales: 2021. www.ons.gov.uk/peoplepopulationandcommunity/birthsdeathsand marriages/livebirths/datasets/birthcharacteristicsinenglandandwales (accessed 13 September 2024).

2 National Centre for Health Statistics. Multiple Births. Data for 2021. www .cdc.gov/nchs/fastats/multiple.htm (accessed 13 September 2024).

3 Boyle, B, McConkey, R, Garne, E, et al. Trends in the prevalence, risk and pregnancy outcome of multiple births with congenital anomaly: a registry-based study in 14 European countries 1984–2007. BJOG. 2013; 120: 707–16.

4 Monden, C, Pison, G, Smits, J. Twin peaks: more twinning in humans than ever before. Hum Reprod. 2021; 36: 1666–73.

5 Gill, P, Lende, MN, van Hook, JW. Twin Births. Treasure Island, FL: StatPearls Publishing, 2023.

6 Hall, JG. Twinning. Lancet. 2003; 362: 735–43.

7 Martin, JA, Hamilton, BE, Ventura, SJ, et al. Births: final data for 2009. Natl Vital Rep. 2011; 60: 1–70.

8 One Child at a Time, Reducing Multiple Births after IVF. Report of the Expert Group on Multiple Births after IVF. https://ifqlive.blob.core.win dows.net/umbraco-website/1311/one-child-at-a-time-report.pdf (accessed 13 September 2024).

9 Human Fertilisation and Embryology Authority. Multiple Births in Fertility Treatment 2019. www.hfea.gov.uk/about-us/publications/research-and-data/ multiple-births-in-fertility-treatment-2019/ (accessed 13 September 2024).

10 Weber, MA, Sebire, NJ. Genetics and developmental pathology of twinning. Semin Fetal Neonatal Med. 2010; 15: 313–18.

11 Benirschke, K, Kim, CK. Multiple pregnancy. 2. N Engl J Med. 1973; 288: 1329–36.

12 Binstock, A, Bodnar, LM, Himes, KP. Severe maternal morbidity in twins. Am J Perinatol. 2023; 40(7): 704–10. http://dx.doi.org/10.1055/a-1974-4449.

13 Witteveen, T, van den Akker, T, Zwart, JJ, Bloemankamp, KW, Roosmalen, JV. Severe acute maternal morbidity in multiple pregnancies: a nationwide cohort study. Am J Obstet Gynecol. 2016; 214(5): 641.e1–e10.

14 Santana, SD, Cecatti, GJ, Surita, FG, et al. Twin pregnancy and severe maternal outcomes: the World Health Organization Multicountry Survey on Maternal and Newborn Health. Obstet Gynecol. 2016; 127(4): 631–41.

15 Nurmi, M, Rautava, P, Gissler, M, Vahlberg, T, Polo-Kantola, P. Incidence and risk factors of hyperemesis gravidarum: a national register-based study in Finland 2005–2017. Acta Obstet Gynecol Scand. 2020; 99(8): 1003–13.

16 Shinar, S, Shapira, U, Maslovitz, S. Redefining normal hemoglobin and anemia in singleton and twin pregnancies. Int J Gynaecol Obstet. 2018; 142: 42–7.

17 Johnson, CY, Rocheleau, CM, Howley, MM, et al. Characteristics of women with urinary tract infection in pregnancy. J Womens Health (Larchmt). 2021; 30: 1556–64.

18 Sibai, BM, Hauth, J, Caritis, S, et al. Hypertensive disorders in twin versus singleton gestations. National Institute of Child Health and Human Development Network of Maternal-Fetal Medicine Units. Am J Obstet Gynecol. 2000; 182: 938–42.

19 Lynch, A, McDuffie, R, Jr, Murphy, J, Faber, K, Orleans, M. Preeclampsia in multiple gestation: the role of assisted reproductive technologies. Obstet Gynecol. 2002; 99: 445–51.

20 Narang, K, Szymanski, LM. Multiple gestations and hypertensive disorders of pregnancy: what do we know? Curr Hypertens Rep. 2020; 23: 1.

21 Gortazar, L, Flores-Le Roux, JA, Benaiges, D, et al. Trends in prevalence of diabetes among twin pregnancies and perinatal outcomes in Catalonia between 2006 and 2015: the DIAGESTCAT study. J Clin Med. 2021; 10: 1937.

22 Liu, X, Landon, MB, Chen, Y, Cheng, W. Perinatal outcomes with intrahepatic cholestasis of pregnancy in twin pregnancies. J Matern Fetal Neonatal Med. 2016; 29: 2176–81.

23 di Marco, G, Bevilacqua, E, Passananti, E, et al. Multiple pregnancy and the risk of postpartum hemorrhage: retrospective analysis in a tertiary level center of care. Diagnostics (Basel). 2023; 13: 446.

24 Fukami, T, Koga, H, Goto, M, et al. Incidence and risk factors for postpartum hemorrhage among transvaginal deliveries at a tertiary perinatal medical facility in Japan. PLoS One. 2019; 14: e0208873.

25 Lapaire, O, Holzgreve, W, Zanetti-Daellenbach, R, et al. Polyhydramnios: an Upd££ate. Donald Sch J Ultrasound Obstet Gynecol. 2007; 1(1): 73–9. http://dx.doi.org/10.5005/jp-journals-10009-1086.

26 Roman, A, Ramirez, A, Fox, NS. Screening for preterm birth in twin pregnancies. Am J Obstet Gynecol MFM. 2022; 4: 100531.

27 Prapas, N, Kalogiannidis, I, Masoura, S, et al. Operative vaginal delivery in singleton term pregnancies: short-term maternal and neonatal outcomes. Hippokratia. 2009; 13: 41–5.

28 Schachter-Safrai, N, Karavani, G, Haj-Yahya, R, Ofek Shlomai, N, Porat, S. Risk factors for cesarean delivery and adverse neonatal outcome in twin pregnancies attempting vaginal delivery. Acta Obstet Gynecol Scand. 2018; 97: 845–51.

29 Hofmeyr, GJ, Barrett, JF, Crowther, CA. Planned cesarean section for women with a twin pregnancy. Cochrane. 2015; 2019: CD006553.

30 Bragg, F, Cromwell, DA, Edozien, LC, et al. Variation in rates of cesarean section among English NHS trusts after accounting for maternal and clinical risk: cross sectional study. BMJ. 2010; 341: c5065.

31 Bradshaw, H, Riddle, JN, Salimgaraev, R, Zhaunova, L, Payne, JL. Risk factors associated with postpartum depressive symptoms: a multinational study. J Affect Disord. 2022; 301: 345–51.

32 Madar, H, Goffinet, F, Seco, A, et al. EPIMOMS (EPIdémiologie de la MOrbidité Maternelle Sévère) study group. Severe acute maternal morbidity in twin compared with singleton pregnancies. Obstet Gynecol. 2019; 133: 1141–50.

33 Jarvis, S, Nelson-Piercy, C. Management of nausea and vomiting in pregnancy. BMJ. 2011; 342: d3606.

34 Einarson, TR, Piwko, C, Koren, G. Quantifying the global rates of nausea and vomiting of pregnancy: a meta analysis. J Popul Ther Clin Pharmacol. 2013; 20: e171–83.

35 Fiaschi, L, Nlson-Piercy, C, Tata, LJ. Hospital admission for hyperemesis gravidarum: a nationwide study of occurrence, reoccurrence and risk factors among 8.2 million pregnancies. Human Repro. 2016; 31(8): 1675–84.

36 Mitsuda, N, Eitoku, M, Maeda, N, Fujieda, M, Suganuma, N. Severity of nausea and vomiting in singleton and twin pregnancies in relation to fetal sex: the Japan Environment and Children's Study (JECS). J Epidemiol. 2019; 29: 340–6.

37 Rao, A, Sairam, S, Shehata, H. Obstetric complications of twin pregnancies. Best Pract Res Clin Obstet Gynaecol. 2004; 18: 557–76.

38 Francisco, C, Gamito, M, Reddy, M, Rolnik, DL. Screening for preeclampsia in twin pregnancies. Best Pract Res Clin Obstet Gynaecol. 2022; 84: 55–65.

39 Day, MC, Barton, JR, O'Brien, JM, Istwan, NB, Sibai, BM. The effect of fetal number on the development of hypertensive conditions of pregnancy. Obstet Gynecol. 2005; 106(5 Pt 1): 927–31.

40 Henry, DE, McElrath, TF, Smith, NA. Preterm severe preeclampsia in singleton and twin pregnancies. J Perinatol 2013; 33(2): 94–7.

41 Wen, SW, Demissie, K, Yang, Q, Walker, MC. Maternal morbidity and obstetric complications in triplet pregnancies and quadruplet and higher-order multiple pregnancies. Am J Obstet Gynecol. 2004; 191(1): 254–8.

42 Yuan, T, Wang, W, Li, XL, et al. Clinical characteristics of fetal and neonatal outcomes in twin pregnancy with preeclampsia in a retrospective case-control study: a STROBE-compliant article. Medicine (Baltim). 2016; 95: e5199.

43 Gonzalez, MC, Reyes, H, Arrese, M, et al. Intrahepatic cholestasis of pregnancy in twin pregnancies. J Hepatol. 1989; 9: 84–90.

44 Feng, C, Li, WJ, He, RH, et al. Impacts of different methods of conception on the perinatal outcome of intrahepatic cholestasis of pregnancy in twin pregnancies. Scientific Reports. 2018; 8: 3985.

45 Weis, MA, Harper, ML, Roehl, KA, Odibo, AO, Cahill, AG. Natural history of placenta previa in twins. Obstet Gynecol. 2012; 120(4): 753–8. http://dx.doi.org/10.1097/AOG.0b013e318269baac.

46 Liu, N, Hu, Q, Liao, H, Wang, X, Yu, H. Vasa previa: perinatal outcomes in singleton and multiple pregnancies. Biosci Trends. 2021; 15: 118–25.

47 Hamza, A, Herr, D, Solomayer, EF, Meyberg-Solomayer, G. Polyhydramnios: causes, diagnosis and therapy. Geburtshilfe Frauenheilkd. 2013; 73: 1241–6.

48 Goldenberg, RL, Culhane, JF, Iams, JD, Romero, R. Epidemiology and causes of preterm birth. Lancet. 2008; 371: 75–84.

49 Chawanpaiboon, S, Vogel, JP, Moller, AB, et al. Global, regional, and national estimates of levels of preterm birth in 2014: a systematic review and modelling analysis. Lancet Glob Health. 2019; 7: e37–e46.

50 Blondel, B, Macfarlane, A, Gissler, M, Breart, G, Zeitlin, J. General obstetrics: preterm birth and multiple pregnancy in European countries participating in the PERISTAT project. BJOG. 2006; 113: 528–35.

51 Victoria, A, Mora, G, Arias, F. Perinatal outcome, placental pathology, and severity of discordance in monochorionic and dichorionic twins. Obstet Gynecol. 2001; 97: 310–15.

52 Bateni, ZH, Clark, SL, Sangi-Haghpeykar, H, et al. Trends in the delivery route of twin pregnancies in the United States, 2006–2013. Eur J Obstet Gynecol Reprod Biol. 2016; 205: 120–6.

53 Ross, LE, McQueen, K, Vigod, S, Dennis, CL. Risk for postpartum depression associated with assisted reproductive technologies and multiple births: a systematic review. Hum Reprod Update. 2011; 17: 96–106.

54 National Institute for Health and Clinical Excellence (NICE). Twin and Triplet Pregnancy. NICE clinical guideline. London: NICE, 2024. www.nice.org.uk/guidance/ng137 (accessed 22nd October 2024).

55 Naert, MN, Khadraoui, H, Muniz Rodriguez, A, Fox, NS. Stratified risk of pregnancy loss for women with a viable singleton pregnancy in the first trimester. J Matern Fetal Neonatal Med. 2022; 35: 4491–5.

56 Batsry, L, Yinon, Y. The vanishing twin: diagnosis and implications. Best Pract Res Clin Obstet Gynaecol. 2022; 84: 66–75.

57 Royal College of Obstetricians and Gynecologists (RCOG). Late Intrauterine Fetal Death and Stillbirth. Green-top guideline no. 55. London: RCOG, 2010.

58 Mackie, FL, Rigby, A, Morris, RK, Kilby, MD. Prognosis of the co-twin following spontaneous single intrauterine fetal death in twin pregnancies: a systematic review and meta-analysis. BJOG. 2019; 126: 569–78.

59 Filipecka-Tyczka, D, Jakiel, G, Kajdy, A, Rabijewski, M. Is growth restriction in twin pregnancies a double challenge? – A narrative review. J Mother Child. 2021; 24: 24–30.

60 Royal College of Obstetricians and Gynecologists (RCOG). Umbilical Cord Prolapse. Green-top guideline no. 50. London: RCOG, 2014.

61 Asahina, R, Tsuda, H, Nishiko, Y, et al. Evaluation of the risk of umbilical cord prolapse in the second twin during vaginal delivery: a retrospective cohort study. BMJ Open. 2021; 11: e046616.

62 Fessehaye, A, Abubeker, F, Daba, M. Locked twins – remote from term: a case report. 2021; 15: 115.

63 Pharoah, PO, Cooke, T. Cerebral palsy and multiple births. Arch Dis Child Fetal Neonatal Ed. 1996; 75: F174–7.

64 Sellier, E, Goldsmith, S, McIntyre, S, et al. Surveillance of Cerebral Palsy Europe Group and the Australian Cerebral Palsy Register Group. Cerebral palsy in twins and higher multiple births: a Europe-Australia population-based study. Dev Med Child Neurol. 2021; 63: 712–20.

65 Draper, ES, Gallimore, ID, Smith, LK, et al. MBRRACE-UK Perinatal Mortality Surveillance Report, UK Perinatal Deaths for Births from January to December 2020. Leicester: The Infant Mortality and Morbidity Studies, Department of Health Sciences, University of Leicester, 2022.

66 Glinianaia, SV, Rankin, J, Wright, C. Congenital anomalies in twins: a register-based study. Hum Reprod. 2008; 23: 1306–11.

67 Lewi, L, Jani, J, Blickstein, I, et al. The outcome of monochorionic diamniotic twin gestations in the era of invasive fetal therapy: a prospective cohort study. Am J Obstet Gynecol. 2008; 199: 514.e1–8.

68 Baxi, LV, Walsh, CA. Monoamniotic twins in contemporary practice: a single-center study of perinatal outcomes. J Matern Fetal Neonatal Med. 2010; 23: 506–10.

69 Jung, YM, Lee, SM, Oh, S, et al. The concordance rate of non-chromosomal congenital malformations in twins based on zygosity: a retrospective cohort study. BJOG. 2021; 128: 857–64.

70 Sperling, L, Kiil, C, Larsen, LU, et al. Detection of chromosal abnormalities, congenital abnormalities and transfusion syndrome in twins. Ultrasoun Obs Gynecol. 2007; 29(5): 517–26.

71 Piro, E, Schierz, IAM, Serra, G, et al. Growth patterns and associated risk factors of congenital malformations in twins. Ital J Pediatr. 2020; 46: 73.

72 Sun, LM, Chen, XK, Wen, SW, et al. Perinatal outcomes of normal cotwins in twin pregnancies with one structurally anomalous fetus: a population-based retrospective study. Am J Perinatol. 2009; 26: 51–6.

73 d'Antonio, F, Khalil, A. Screening and diagnosis of chromosomal abnormalities in twin pregnancy. Best Pract Res Clin Obstet Gynaecol. 2022; 84: 229–39.

74 The Fetal Medicine Foundation. Structural Abnormalities. https://fetalmedi cine.org/education/fetal-abnormalities/multiple-pregnancies/structural-abnormalities (accessed 15 September 2024).

75 Wen, SW, Miao, Q, Taljaard, M, et al. Associations of assisted reproductive technology and twin pregnancy with risk of congenital heart defects. JAMA Pediatr. 2020; 174: 446–54.

76 Zamani, Z, Parekh, U. Vanishing Twin Syndrome. Treasure Island, FL: StatPearls Publishing, 2022.

77 Harris, AL, Sacha, CR, Basnet, KM, et al. Vanishing twins conceived through fresh in vitro fertilization: obstetric outcomes and placental pathology. Obstet Gynecol. 2020; 135: 1426–33.

78 Kamath, MS, Antonisamy, B, Selliah, HY, Sunkara, SK. Perinatal outcomes of singleton live births with and without vanishing twin following transfer of multiple embryos: analysis of 113 784 singleton live births. Hum Reprod. 2018; 33: 2018–22.

79 d'Antonio, F, Khalil, A, Dias, T, Thilaganathan, B. Early fetal loss in monochorionic and dichorionic twin pregnancies: analysis of the Southwest Thames Obstetric Research Collaborative (STORK) multiple pregnancy cohort. Ultrasound Obstet Gynecol. 2013; 41: 632–6.

80 Sebire, NJ, Thornton, S, Hughes, K, Snijders, RJ, Nicolaides, KH. The prevalence and consequences of missed abortion in twin pregnancies at 10 to 14 weeks of gestation. Br J Obstet Gynaecol. 1997; 104: 847–8.

81 Morris, RK, Mackie, F, Garces, AT, Knight, M, Kilby, MD. The incidence, maternal, fetal and neonatal consequences of single intrauterine fetal death in monochorionic twins: a prospective observational UKOSS study. PLoS One. 2020; 15: e0239477.

82 Hillman, SC, Morris, RK, Kilby, MD. Co-twin prognosis after single fetal death: a systematic review and meta-analysis. Obstet Gynecol. 2011; 118: 928–40.

83 Morin, L, Lim, K, Bly, S, et al. Ultrasound in twin pregnancies: no. 260, June 2011. Int J Gynecol Obstet. 2011; 115: 117–18.

84 Breathnach, FM, Malone, FD. Fetal growth disorders in twin gestations. Semin Perinatol. 2012; 36: 175–81.

85 Hirsch, L, Okby, R, Freeman, H, et al. Differences in fetal growth patterns between twins and singletons. J Matern Fetal Neonatal Med. 2020; 33(15): 2546–55. http://dx.doi.org/10.1080/14767058.2018.1555705.

86 Cerra, C, d'Antonio, F. Discordance in twins: association versus prediction. Best Pract Res Clin Obstet Gynaecol. 2022; 84: 33–42.

87 Kalafat, E, Thilaganathan, B, Papageorghiou, A, Bhide, A, Khalil, A. Significance of placental cord insertion site in twin pregnancy. Ultrasound Obstet Gynecol. 2018; 52: 378–84.

88 Couck, I, Mourad Tawfic, N, Deprest, J, et al. Does site of cord insertion increase risk of adverse outcome, twin-to-twin transfusion syndrome and discordant growth in monochorionic twin pregnancy? Ultrasound Obstet Gynecol. 2018; 52: 385–9.

89 Khalil, A, Beune, I, Hecher, K, et al. Consensus definition and essential reporting parameters of selective fetal growth restriction in twin pregnancy: a Delphi procedure. Ultrasound Obstet Gynecol. 2019; 53: 47–54.

90 d'Antonio, F, Odibo, AO, Prefumo, F, Khalil, A, Buca, Flacco, ME. Weight discordance and perinatal mortality in twin pregnancy: systematic review and meta-analysis. Ultrasound Obstet Gynecol. 2018; 52: 11–23.

91 Breathnach, FM, McAuliffe, FM, Geary, M, et al. Definition of intertwin birth weight discordance. Obstet Gynecol. 2011; 118: 94–103.

92 Khalil, A, Rodgers, M, Baschat, A, et al. ISUOG practice guidelines: role of ultrasound in twin pregnancy. Ultrasound Obstet Gynecol. 2016; 47: 247–63.

93 American College of Obstetricians and Gynecologists' Committee on Practice Bulletins – Obstetrics; Society for Maternal–Fetal Medicine. Practice bulletin No. 169: multifetal gestations: twin, triplet, and higher-order multifetal pregnancies. Obstet Gynecol. 2016; 128: e131–46.

94 The Fetal Medicine Foundation. MC Twins: Selective Fetal Growth Restriction. https://fetalmedicine.org/education/fetal-abnormalities/mul tiple-pregnancies/mc-twins-selective-fetal-growth-restriction (accessed 15 September 2024).

95 Royal College of Obstetricians and Gynaecologists (RCOG). Management of Monochorionic Twin Pregnancy, 2nd edn. Green-top guideline no. 51. London: RCOG, 2016. www.rcog.org.uk/en/guidelines-research-services/ guidelines/gtg51/ (accessed 15 September 2024).

96 di Mascio, D, Acharya, G, Khalil, A, et al. Birthweight discordance and neonatal morbidity in twin pregnancies: a systematic review and meta-analysis. Acta Obstet Gynecol Scand. 2019; 98: 1245–57.

97 Khalil, A, Prasad, S. Screening and prevention of preterm birth in twin pregnancies. Best Pract Res Clin Obstet Gynaecol. 2022; 84: 179–93.

98 Ananth, CV, Joseph, K, Demissie, K, Vintzileos, AM. Trends in twin preterm birth subtypes in the United States, 1989 through 2000: impact on perinatal mortality. Am J Obstet Gynecol. 2005; 193: e1–9.

99 Murray, S, Stock, S, Coman, S, Cooper, E, Norman, J. Spontaneous preterm birth prevention in multiple pregnancy. Obstet Gynaecol. 2018; 20: 57–63.

100 Breathnach, FM, McAuliffe, FM, Geary, M, et al. Perinatal Ireland Research Consortium. Optimum timing for planned delivery of uncomplicated monochorionic and dichorionic twin pregnancies. Obstet Gynecol. 2012; 119: 50–9.

101 Marleen, S, Dias, C, Nandasena, R, et al. Association between chorionicity and preterm birth in twin pregnancies: a systematic review involving 29 864 twin pregnancies. BJOG. 2021; 128: 788–96.

102 Borah, T, Das, A. Locked twins: a rarity. Ann Med Health Sci Res. 2012; 2: 204–5.

103 Khalil, A, Bhide, AT, Papageorghiou, A, Thilaganathan, B. Reduction in twin stillbirth following implementation of NICE guidance. Ultrasound Obstet Gynecol. 2020; 56: 566–71.

104 Draper, ES, Gallimore, ID, Kurinczuk, JJ, Kenyon, S (eds.) on behalf of MBRRACE-UK. MBRRACE-UK 2019 Perinatal Confidential Enquiry: Stillbirths and Neonatal Deaths in Twin Pregnancies. Leicester: The Infant Mortality and Morbidity Studies, Department of Health Sciences, University of Leicester, 2021.

105 Dube, J, Dodds, L, Armson, BA. Does chorionicity or zygosity predict adverse perinatal outcomes in twins? Am J Obstet Gynecol. 2002; 186: 579–83.

106 Danon, D, Sekar, R, Hack, KE, Fisk, NM. Increased stillbirth in uncomplicated monochorionic twin pregnancies: a systematic review and meta-analysis. Obstet Gynecol. 2013; 121: 1318–26.

107 d'Antonio, F, Odibo, A, Berghella, V, et al. Perinatal mortality, timing of delivery and prenatal management of monoamniotic twin pregnancy: systematic review and meta-analysis. Ultrasound Obstet Gynecol. 2019; 53: 166–74.

108 Mutchinick, OM, Luna-Muñoz, L, Amar, E, et al. Conjoined twins: a worldwide collaborative epidemiological study of the International Clearinghouse for Birth Defects Surveillance and Research. Am J Med Genet C Semin Med Genet. 2011; 157: 274–87.

109 Glinianaia, SV, Rankin, J, Khalil, A, et al. Prevalence, antenatal management and perinatal outcome of monochorionic monoamniotic twin pregnancy:

a collaborative multicenter study in England, 2000–2013. Ultrasound Obstet Gynecol. 2019; 53: 184–92.

110 Chauhan, SP, Scardo, JA, Hayes, E, et al. Twins: prevalence, problems, and preterm births. Am J Obstet Gynecol. 2010; 203: 305–15.

111 Lewi, L, Valencia, C, Gonzalez, E, Deprest, J, Nicolaides, KH. The outcome of twin reversed arterial perfusion sequence diagnosed in the first trimester. Am J Obstet Gynecol. 2010; 203: 213.e1–4.

112 Bamberg, C, Hecher, K. Twin-to-twin transfusion syndrome: controversies in the diagnosis and management. Best Pract Res Clin Obstet Gynaecol. 2022; 84: 143–54.

113 Nicholas, L, Fischbein, R, Ernst-Milner, S, Wani, R. Review of international clinical guidelines related to prenatal screening during monochorionic pregnancies. J Clin Med. 2021; 10: 1128–47.

114 Spitz, L. Conjoined twins. Br J Surg. 1996; 83(8): 1028–30.

115 Mian, A, Gabra, NI, Sharma, T, et al. Conjoined twins: from conception to separation, a review. Clin Anat. 2017; 30: 385–96.

116 Chen, CP, Hsu, CY, Su, JW, et al. Conjoined twins detected in the first trimester: a review. Taiwan J Obstet Gynecol. 2011; 50: 424–31.

117 van Mieghem T, Abbasi N, Shinar S, et al. Monochorionic monoamniotic twin pregnancies. Am J Obstet Gynecol MFM. 2022; 4: 100520.

118 Rossi, AC, Prefumo, F. Impact of cord entanglement on perinatal outcome of monoamniotic twins: a systematic review of the literature. Ultrasound Obstet Gynecol. 2013; 41: 131–5.

119 Sueters, M, Oepkes, D. Diagnosis of twin-to-twin transfusion syndrome, selective fetal growth restriction, twin–polycythemia sequence, and twin reversed arterial perfusion sequence. Best Pract Res Clin Obstet Gynaecol. 2014; 28: 215–26.

120 Badr, DA, Carlin, A, Kang, X, et al. Evaluation of the new expert consensus-based definition of selective fetal growth restriction in monochorionic pregnancies. J Matern Fetal Neonatal Med. 2022; 35: 2338–44.

121 Gratacos, E, Lewi, L, Muñoz, B, et al. A classification system for selective intrauterine growth restriction in monochorionic pregnancies according to umbilical artery Doppler flow in the smaller twin. Ultrasound Obstet Gynecol. 2007; 30: 28–34.

122 Gratacos, E, Antolin, E, Lewi, L, et al. Monochorionic twins with selective intrauterine growth restriction and intermittent absent or reversed end-diastolic flow (Type III): feasibility and perinatal outcome of fetoscopic placental laser coagulation. Ultrasound Obstet Gynecol. 2008; 31: 669–75.

123 van Gemert, MJC, van den Wijngaard, JPHM, Vandenbussche, FPHA. Twin reversed arterial perfusion sequence is more common than generally accepted. Birth Defects Res a Clin Mol Teratol. 2015; 103(7): 641–3. http://dx.doi.org/10.1002/bdra.23405.

124 Quintero, RA, Morales, WJ, Allen, MH, et al. Staging of twin–twin transfusion syndrome. J Perinatol. 1999; 19: 550–5.

125 Hecher, K, Gardiner, HM, Diemert, A, Bartmann, P. Long-term outcomes for monochorionic twins after laser therapy in twin-to-twin transfusion syndrome. Lancet Child Adolesc Health. 2018; 2: 525–35.

126 Lopriore, E, Oepkes, D, Walther, FJ. Neonatal morbidity in twin–twin transfusion syndrome. Early Hum Dev. 2011; 87: 595–9.

127 Tollenaar, LSA, Slaghekke, F, Lewi, L, et al. Spontaneous twin anemia polycythemia sequence: diagnosis, management, and outcome in an international cohort of 249 cases. Am J Obstet Gynecol. 2021; 224: e1–213.

128 Assaf, SA, Benirschke, K, Chmait, RH. Spontaneous twin anemia–polycythemia sequence complicated by recipient placental vascular thrombosis and hydrops fetalis. J Matern Fetal Neonatal Med. 2011; 24: 549–52.

129 Slaghekke, F, Kist, WJ, Oepkes, D, et al. Twin anemia–polycythemia sequence: diagnostic criteria, classification, perinatal management and outcome. Fetal Diagn Ther. 2010; 27: 181–90.

130 Murray, SR, Norman, JE. Multiple pregnancies following assisted reproductive technologies – a happy consequence or double trouble? Semin Fetal Neonatal Med. 2014; 19: 222–7.

131 Practice Committee of the American Society for Reproductive Medicine, Practice Committee of the Society for Assisted Reproductive Technologies. Guidance on the limits to the number of embryos to transfer: a committee opinion. Fertil Steril. 2017; 107: 901–3.

132 Bai, F, Wang, DY, Fan, YJ, et al. Assisted reproductive technology service availability, efficacy and safety in mainland China: 2016. Hum Reprod. 2020; 35: 446–52.

133 Adamson, GD, Normal, RJ. Why are multiple pregnancy rates and single embryo transfer rates so different globally, and what do we do about it? Fertil Steril. 2020; 114(4): 680–9.

134 Kamath, MS, Mascarenhas, M, Kirubakaran, R, Bhattacharya, S. Number of embryos for transfer following in vitro fertilisation or intra-cytoplasmic sperm injection. Cochrane Database Syst Rev. 2020; (8): CD003416.

135 Ma, S, Peng, Y, Hu, L, et al. Comparisons of benefits and risks of single embryo transfer versus double embryo transfer: a systematic review and meta-analysis. Reprod Biol Endocrinol. 2022; 20: 20.

136 Luke, B, Gopal, D, Cabral, H, et al. Adverse pregnancy, birth, and infant outcomes in twins: effects of maternal fertility status and infant gender combinations; the Massachusetts Outcomes Study of Assisted Reproductive Technology. Am J Obstet Gynecol. 2017; 217: 330.e1–15. http://dx.doi.org/10.1016/j.ajog.2017.04.025.

137 Glujovsky, D, Retamar, AMQ, Sedo, CRA, et al. Cleavage stage versus blastocyst stage embryo transfer in assisted reproductive technology. Cochrane Database Syst Rev. 2022; (5): CD002118.

138 Busnelli, A, Dallagiovanna, C, Reschini, M, et al. Risk factors for mono-zygotic twinning after in vitro fertilization: a systematic review and meta-analysis. Fertil Steril. 2019; 111: 302–17.

139 Ellings, JM, Newman, RB, Hulsey, TC, Bivins, HA, Keenan, A. Reduction in very low birth weight deliveries and perinatal mortality in a specialized, multidisciplinary twin clinic. Obstet Gynecol. 1993; 81: 387–91.

140 Newman, RB, Ellings, JM. Antepartum management of the multiple gestation: the case for specialized care. Semin Perinatol. 1995; 19: 387–403.

141 Ruk, RJ, Brown, CE, Peters, MT, Johnston, AB. Specialized care for twin gestations: improving newborn outcomes und reducing costs. J Obstet Gynecol Neonatal Nurs. 2001; 30: 52–60.

142 National Institute for Health and Care Excellence (NICE). Multiple Pregnancy: Twin and Triplet Pregnancies. NICE Quality Standard QS 46. London: NICE, 2013 (updated September 2019). www.nice.org.uk/guidance/qs46 (accessed 15 September 2024).

143 Twins and Multiple Births Association (TAMBA). NICE Works: Twins and Multiple Births Association Maternity Engagement Project Final Report. Aldershot: TAMBA, 2019. https://twinstrust.org/static/fc9b2326-a70f-4989-b64b3cafe05f3440/NICE-works-final-report.pdf (accessed 1 October 2024).

144 Bricker, L, Reed, K, Wood, L, Neilson, JP. Nutritional advice for improving outcomes in multiple pregnancies. Cochrane Database Syst Rev. 2015; (11): CD008867.

145 National Institute for Health and Care Excellence (NICE). Antenatal Care. NICE Clinical Guideline NG201. London: NICE, 2021. www.nice.org.uk/guidance/ng201 (accessed 15 September 2024).

146 Norwitz, ER, Edusa, V, Shin Park, J. Maternal physiology and complications of multiple pregnancy. Semin Perinatol. 2005; 29(5): 338–48. http://dx.doi.org/10.1053/j.semperi.2005.08.002.

147 Stock, S, Norman, J. Preterm and term labour in multiple pregnancies. Seminars Fetal Neonatal Med. 2010; 15(6): 336–41.

148 National Institute for Health and Care Excellence (NICE). Preterm Labour and Birth. NICE Guideline NG25. London: NICE, 2022. www.nice.org.uk/ guidance/ng25 (accessed 15 September 2024).

149 dos Santos, F, Daru, J, Rogozińska, E, Cooper, NAM. Accuracy of fetal fibronectin for assessing preterm birth risk in asymptomatic pregnant women: a systematic review and meta-analysis. Acta Obstet Gynecol Scand. 2018; 97: 657–67.

150 Kuhrt, K, Hezelgrave-Elliott, N, Stock, SJ, et al. Quantitative fetal fibro-nectin for prediction of preterm birth in asymptomatic twin pregnancy. Acta Obstet Gynecol Scand. 2020; 99: 1191–7.

151 Carter, J, Seed, PT, Watson, HA, et al. Development and validation of predictive models for QUiPP App v.2: tool for predicting preterm birth in women with symptoms of threatened preterm labor. Ultrasound Obstet Gynecol. 2020; 55: 357–67.

152 Singer, E, Pilpel, S, Bsat, F, et al. Accuracy of fetal fibronectin to predict preterm birth in twin gestations with symptoms of labor. Obstet Gynecol. 2007; 109: 1083–7.

153 Kindinger, L, Poon, L, Cacciatore, S, et al. The effect of gestational age and cervical length measurements in the prediction of spontaneous preterm birth in twin pregnancies: an individual patient level meta-analysis. BJOG. 2016; 123: 877–84.

154 American College of Obstetricians and Gynecologists' Committee on Practice Bulletins – Obstetrics; Society for Maternal–Fetal Medicine. Multifetal gestations: twin, triplet, and higher-order multifetal pregnan-cies: ACOG practice bulletin, number 231. Obstet Gynecol. 2021; 137: e145–62.

155 SMFM Research Committee ; Grantz, KL, Kawakita, T, Lu, YL, et al. SMFM special statement: state of the science on multifetal gestations: unique considerations and importance. Am J Obstet Gynecol. 2019; 221: B2–12.

156 da Silva Lopes, K, Takemoto, Y, Ota, E, Tanigaki, S, Mori, R. Bed rest with and without hospitalisation in multiple pregnancy for improving perinatal outcomes. Cochrane Database Syst Rev. 2017; (3): CD012031.

157 Dodd, JM, Grivell, RM, O'Brien, CM, Dowswell, T, Deussen, AR. Prenatal administration of progestogens for preventing spontaneous pre-term birth in women with a multiple pregnancy. Cochrane Database Syst Rev. 2019; (11): CD012024.

158 Romero, R, Conde-Agudelo, A, El-Refaie, W, et al. Vaginal progesterone decreases preterm birth and neonatal morbidity and mortality in women with a twin gestation and a short cervix: an updated meta-analysis of individual patient data. Ultrasound Obstet Gynecol. 2017; 49: 303–14.

159 El-Refaie, W, Abdelhafez, MS, Badawy, A. Vaginal progesterone for prevention of preterm labor in asymptomatic twin pregnancies with sonographic short cervix: a randomized clinical trial of efficacy and safety. Arch Gynecol Obstet. 2016; 293: 61–7.

160 American College of Obstetricians and Gynecologists' Committee on Practice Bulletins – Obstetrics. Prediction and prevention of spontaneous preterm birth: ACOG practice bulletin, number 234. Obstet Gynecol. 2021; 138: e65–90.

161 Royal Australian and New Zealand College of Obstericians and Gynaecologists (RANZCOG). Progesterone: Use in the Second and Third Trimester of Pregnancy for the Prevention of Preterm Birth. Best practice statement. Melbourne: RANZCOG, 2017.

162 EPPPIC Group. Evaluating Progestogens for Preventing Preterm birth International Collaborative (EPPPIC): meta-analysis of individual participant data from randomised controlled trials. Lancet. 2021; 397: 1183–94.

163 Rehal, A, Benkő, Z, De Paco Matallana, C, et al. Early vaginal progesterone versus placebo in twin pregnancies for the prevention of spontaneous preterm birth: a randomized, double-blind trial. Am J Obstet Gynecol. 2021; 224: 86.e1–19.

164 Romero, R, Conde-Agudelo, A, Rehal, A, et al. Vaginal progesterone for the prevention of preterm birth and adverse perinatal outcomes in twin gestations with a short cervix: an updated individual patient data meta-analysis. Ultrasound Obstet Gynecol. 2022; 59: 263–6.

165 The George Washington University Biostatistics Center. A trial of pessary and progesterone for preterm prevention in twin gestation with a short cervix. clinicaltrials.gov. 2021. Report No.: NCT02518594. https://clini caltrials.gov/ct2/show/NCT02518594 (accessed 15 September 2024).

166 ISUOG. Role of ultrasound in the prediction of spontaneous preterm birth. www.isuog.org/resource/practice-guidelines-preterm-birth-pdf.html (accessed 15 September 2024).

167 Liem, SM, van Pampus, MG, Mol, BW, Bekedam, DJ. Cervical pessaries for the prevention of preterm birth: a systematic review. Obstet Gynecol Int. 2013; 2013: 576723.

168 Liem, S, Schuit, E, Hegeman, M, et al. Cervical pessaries for prevention of preterm birth in women with a multiple pregnancy (ProTWIN): a multicentre, open-label randomised controlled trial. Lancet. 2013; 382: 1341–9.

169 Goya, M, de la Calle, M, Pratcorona, L, et al. Cervical pessary to prevent preterm birth in women with twin gestation and sonographic short cervix:

a multicenter randomized controlled trial (PECEP-Twins). Am J Obstet Gynecol. 2016; 214: 145–52.

170 Nicolaides, KH, Syngelaki, A, Poon, LC, et al. Cervical pessary placement for prevention of preterm birth in unselected twin pregnancies: a randomized controlled trial. Am J Obstet Gynecol. 2016; 214: 3.e1–9.

171 Pratcorona, L, Goya, M, Merced, C, et al. Cervical pessary to reduce preterm birth <34 weeks of gestation after an episode of preterm labor and a short cervix: a randomized controlled trial. Am J Obstet Gynecol. 2018; 219: 99.e1–16.

172 Thangatorai, R, Lim, FC, Nalliah, S. Cervical pessary in the prevention of preterm births in multiple pregnancies with a short cervix: PRISMA compliant systematic review and meta-analysis. J Matern Fetal Neonatal Med. 2018; 31: 1638–45.

173 Norman, JE, Norrie, J, MacLennan, G, et al. Evaluation of the Arabin cervical pessary for prevention of preterm birth in women with a twin pregnancy and short cervix (STOPPIT-2): an open-label randomised trial and updated meta-analysis. PLoS Med. 2021; 18: e1003506.

174 Rafael, TJ, Berghella, V, Alfirevic, Z. Cervical stitch (cerclage) for preventing preterm birth in multiple pregnancy. Cochrane Database Syst Rev. 2014; (9): CD009166.

175 Rottenstreich, A, Levin, G, Kleinstern, G, et al. History-indicated cervical cerclage in management of twin pregnancy. Ultrasound Obstet Gynecol. 2019; 54: 517–23.

176 Li, C, Shen, J, Hua, K. Cerclage for women with twin pregnancies: a systematic review and metaanalysis. Am J Obstet Gynecol. 2019; 220: 543–57.

177 Atia, H. Prophylactic cerclage for twin pregnancy with shortened cervix. clinicaltrials.gov. 2022. Report No.: NCT05338164. https://clinicaltrials.gov/ct2/show/NCT05338164 (accessed 15 September 2024).

178 Lv, MD. Cerclage for short cervix in twins. clinicaltrials.gov. 2018. Report No.: NCT02912390. https://clinicaltrials.gov/ct2/show/NCT02912390 (accessed 15 September 2024).

179 Roman, A, Zork, N, Haeri, S, et al. Physical examination-indicated cerclage in twin pregnancy: a randomized controlled trial. Am J Obstet Gynecol. 2020; 223: 902.e1–e11.

180 Gyamfi, C, Lerner, V, Holzman, I, Stone, JL. Routine cervical length in twins and perinatal outcomes. Am J Perinatol. 2007; 24: 65–9.

181 Palas, D, Ehlinger, V, Alberge, C, et al. Efficacy of antenatal corticosteroids in preterm twins: the EPIPAGE-2 cohort study. BJOG. 2018; 125: 1164–70.

182 Royal College of Obstetricians and Gynaecologists (RCOG). Preterm Prelabor Rupture of the Membranes. Green-top guideline no. 44. London: RCOG, 2010. www.rcog.org.uk/globalassets/documents/guidelines/gtg_44 .pdf (accessed 15 September 2024).

183 Kenyon, S, Brocklehurst, P, Jones, D, et al. MRC ORACLE Children Study. Long term outcomes following prescription of antibiotics to pregnant women with either spontaneous preterm labor or preterm rupture of the membranes. BMC Pregnancy Childbirth. 2008; 8: 14.

184 Sela, HY, Simpson, LL. Preterm premature rupture of membranes complicating twin pregnancy: management considerations. Clin Obstet Gynecol. 2011; 54: 321–9.

185 Doyle, LW, Crowther, CA, Middleton, P, Marret, S, Rouse, D. Magnesium sulphate for women at risk of preterm birth for neuroprotection of the fetus. Cochrane Database Syst Rev. 2009; (1): CD004661.

186 Wilson, A, Hodgetts-Morton, VA, Marson, EJ, et al. Tocolytics for delaying preterm birth: a network meta-analysis (0924). Cochrane Database Syst Rev. 2022; (8): CD014978. http://dx.doi.org/10.1002/ 14651858.CD014978.pub2.

187 Tel-Aviv Sourasky Medical Center. Tocolytic therapy for preterm labor in multiple gestation. clinicaltrials.gov. 2016. Report No.: NCT02725736. https://clinicaltrials.gov/ct2/show/NCT02725736 (accessed 15 September 2024).

188 Cheung, KW, Seto, MTY, Wang, W, et al. Effect of delayed interval delivery of remaining fetus(es) in multiple pregnancies on survival: a systematic review and meta-analysis. Am J Obstet Gynecol. 2020; 222: 306–19.

189 d'Antonio, F, Khalil, A, Pagani, G, et al. Crown-rump length discordance and adverse perinatal outcome in twin pregnancies: systematic review and meta-analysis. Ultrasound Obstet Gynecol. 2014; 44: 138–46.

190 Lewi, L, Lewi, P, Diemert, A, et al. The role of ultrasound examination in the first trimester and at 16 weeks' gestation to predict fetal complications in monochorionic diamniotic twin pregnancies. Am J Obstet Gynecol. 2008; 199: 493.e1–7.

191 Memmo, A, Dias, T, Mahsud-Dornan, S, et al. Prediction of selective fetal growth restriction and twin-to-twin transfusion syndrome in monochorionic twins. BJOG. 2012; 119: 417–21.

192 Kurtz, A, Wapner, R, Mata, J, Johnson, A, Morgan, P. Twin pregnancies: accuracy of first-trimester abdominal US in predicting chorionicity and amnionicity. Radiology. 1992; 185: 759–62.

193 Monteagudo, A, Timor-Tritsch, IE, Sharma, S. Early and simple determination of chorionic and amniotic type in multifetal gestations in the first

fourteen weeks by high-frequency transvaginal ultrasonography. Am J Obstet Gynecol. 1994; 170: 824–9.

194 Lu, J, Ting, YH, Leung, TY. Determining chorionicity and amnionicity in twin pregnancies: pitfalls. Best Pract Res Clin Obstet Gynaecol. 2022; 84: 2–16.

195 Lu, J, Cheng, YKY, Ting, YH, Law, KM, Leung, TY. Pitfalls in assessing chorioamnionicity: novel observations and literature review. Am J Obstet Gynecol. 2018; 219: 242–54.

196 Maruotti, GM, Saccone, G, Morlando, M, Martinelli, P. First-trimester ultrasound determination of chorionicity in twin gestations using the lambda sign: a systematic review and meta-analysis. Eur J Obstet Gynecol Reprod Biol. 2016; 202: 66–70.

197 Sepulveda, W, Sebire, NJ, Hughes, K, Kalogeropoulos, A, Nicolaides, KH. Evolution of the lambda or twin-chorionic peak sign in dichorionic twin pregnancies. Obstet Gynecol. 1997; 89: 439–41.

198 Gueneuc, A, Spaggiari, E, Bonniere, M, et al. Pitfall in the diagnosis of chorionicity in twin pregnancy at first trimester. Ultrasound Obstet Gynecol. 2017; 49: 277–8.

199 Dias, T, Arcangeli, T, Bhide, A, et al. First-trimester ultrasound determination of chorionicity in twin pregnancy. Ultrasound Obstet Gynecol. 2011; 38: 530–2.

200 Fenton, C, Reidy, K, Demyanenko, M, et al. The significance of yolk sac number in monoamniotic twins. Fetal Diagn Ther. 2019; 46: 193–9.

201 Dias, T, Ladd, S, Mahsud-Dornan, S, et al. Systematic labeling of twin pregnancies on ultrasound. Ultrasound Obstet Gynecol. 2011; 38: 130–3.

202 Mackie, FL, Whittle, R, Morris, RK, et al. First-trimester ultrasound measurements and maternal serum biomarkers as prognostic factors in monochorionic twins: a cohort study. Diagn Progn Res. 2019; 3: 9.

203 Prats, P, Rodríguez, I, Comas, C, Puerto, B. Systematic review of screening for trisomy 21 in twin pregnancies in first trimester combining nuchal translucency and biochemical markers: a meta-analysis. Prenat Diagn. 2014; 34: 1077–83.

204 Sarno, L, Revello, R, Hanson, E, Akolekar, R, Nicolaides, KH. Prospective first-trimester screening for trisomies by cell-free DNA testing of maternal blood in twin pregnancy. Ultrasound Obstet Gynecol. 2016; 47: 705–11.

205 Khalil, A, Archer, R, Hutchinson, V, et al. Noninvasive prenatal screening in twin pregnancies with cell-free DNA using the IONA test: a prospective multicenter study. Am J Obstet Gynecol. 2021; 225: 79.e1–13.

206 Revello, R, Sarno, L, Ispas, A, Akolekar, R, Nicolaides, KH. Screening for trisomies by cell-free DNA testing of maternal blood: consequences of a failed result. Ultrasound Obstet Gynecol. 2016; 47(6): 698–704.

207 Leung, TY, Qu, JZ, Liao, GJ, et al. Noninvasive twin zygosity assessment and aneuploidy detection by maternal plasma DNA sequencing. Prenat Diagn. 2013; 33: 675–81.

208 Qu, JZ, Leung, TY, Jiang, P, et al. Noninvasive prenatal determination of twin zygosity by maternal plasma DNA analysis. Clin Chem. 2013; 59: 427–35.

209 Benn, P, Rebarber, A. Non-invasive prenatal testing in the management of twin pregnancies. Prenat Diagn. 2021; 41: 1233–40.

210 Balaguer, N, Mateu-Brull, E, Serra, V, Simón, C, Milán, M. Should vanishing twin pregnancies be systematically excluded from cell-free fetal DNA testing? Prenat Diagn. 2021; 41: 1241–8.

211 Chaveeva, P, Wright, A, Syngelaki, A, et al. First-trimester screening for trisomies in pregnancies with vanishing twin. Ultrasound Obstet Gynecol. 2020; 55: 326–31.

212 Public Health England. NHS fetal anomaly screening programme (FASP): programme overview. www.gov.uk/guidance/fetal-anomaly-screening-programme-overview (accessed 15 September 2024).

213 Palomaki, GE, Chiu, RWK, Pertile, MD, et al. International Society for Prenatal Diagnosis position statement: cell free (cf)DNA screening for Down syndrome in multiple pregnancies. Prenat Diagn. 2021; 41: 1222–32.

214 American College of Obstetricians and Gynecologists' Committee on Practice Bulletins – Obstetrics; Committee on Genetics; Society for Maternal–Fetal Medicine. Screening for fetal chromosomal abnormalities: ACOG practice bulletin, number 226. Obstet Gynecol. 2020; 136: e48–69.

215 di Mascio, D, Khalil, A, Rizzo, G, et al. Risk of fetal loss following amniocentesis or chorionic villus sampling in twin pregnancy: systematic review and meta-analysis. Ultrasound Obstet Gynecol. 2020; 56: 647–55.

216 Gil, MM, Rodríguez-Fernández, M, Elger, T, et al. Risk of fetal loss after chorionic villus sampling in twin pregnancy derived from propensity score matching analysis. Ultrasound Obstet Gynecol. 2022; 59: 162–8.

217 Elger, T, Akolekar, R, Syngelaki, A, et al. Fetal loss after chorionic villus sampling in twin pregnancy. Ultrasound Obstet Gynecol. 2021; 58: 48–55.

218 Antsaklis, A, Daskalakis, G, Souka, AP, Kavalakis, Y, Michalas, S. Fetal blood sampling in twin pregnancies. Ultrasound Obstet Gynecol. 2003; 22: 377–9.

219 Corcoran, S, Breathnach, F, Burke, G, et al. Dichorionic twin ultrasound surveillance: sonography every 4 weeks significantly underperforms sonography every 2 weeks: results of the prospective multicentre ESPRiT study. Am J Obstet Gynecol. 2015; 213: 551.e1–5.

220 The Royal Australian and New Zealand College of Obstericians and Gynaecologists (RANZCOG). Management of Monochorionic Twin Pregnancy. Best practice statement. Melbourne: RANZCOG, 2021.

221 FIGO Working Group on Good Clinical Practice in Maternal–Fetal Medicine. Good clinical practice advice: management of twin pregnancy. Int J Gynaecol Obstet. 2019; 144: 330–7.

222 Khalil, A, d'Antonio, F, Dias, T, Cooper, D, Thilaganathan, B. Southwest Thames Obstetric Research Collaborative (STORK). Ultrasound estimation of birth weight in twin pregnancy: comparison of biometry algorithms in the STORK multiple pregnancy cohort. Ultrasound Obstet Gynecol. 2014; 44: 210–20.

223 Stirrup, OT, Khalil, A, d'Antonio, F, et al. Fetal growth reference ranges in twin pregnancy: analysis of the Southwest Thames Obstetric Research Collaborative (STORK) multiple pregnancy cohort. Ultrasound Obstet Gynecol. 2015; 45(3): 301–7. http://dx.doi.org/10.1002/uog.14640.

224 Odibo, AO, Cahill, AG, Goetzinger, KR, et al. Customized growth charts for twin gestations to optimize identification of small-for-gestational age fetuses at risk of intrauterine fetal death. Ultrasound Obstet Gynecol. 2013; 41(6): 637–42. http://dx.doi.org/10.1002/uog.12404.

225 Kalafat, E, Sebghati, M, Thilaganathan, B, et al. Predictive accuracy of Southwest Thames Obstetric Research Collaborative (STORK) chorionicity-specific twin growth charts for stillbirth: a validation study. Ultrasound Obstet Gynecol. 2019; 53(2): 193–9. http://dx.doi.org/10.1002/uog.19069.

226 Hiersch, L, Barrett, J, Fox, NS, et al. Should twin-specific growth charts be used to assess fetal growth in twin pregnancies? Am J Obstet Gynecol. 2022; 227: 10–28.

227 Koch, AK, Burger, RJ, Schuit, E, et al. Timing of delivery for twins with growth discordance and growth restriction: an individual participant data meta-analysis. Obstet Gynecol. 2022; 139: 1155–67.

228 Valsky, DV, Eixarch, E, Martinez, JM, Crispi, F, Gratacós, E. Selective intrauterine growth restriction in monochorionic twins: pathophysiology, diagnostic approach and management dilemmas. Semin Fetal Neonatal Med. 2010; 15: 342–8.

229 Ishii, K, Murakoshi, T, Takahashi, Y, et al. Perinatal outcome of monochorionic twins with selective intrauterine growth restriction and different

types of umbilical artery Doppler under expectant management. Fetal Diagn Ther. 2009; 26: 157–61.

230 Townsend, R, d'Antonio, F, Sileo, FG, et al. Perinatal outcome of mono-chorionic twin pregnancy complicated by selective fetal growth restriction according to management: systematic review and meta-analysis. Ultrasound Obstet Gynecol. 2019;53(1): 36–46. http://dx.doi.org/10.1002/uog.20114.

231 Monaghan, C, Kalafat, E, Binder, J, Thilaganathan, B, Khalil, A. Prediction of adverse pregnancy outcome in monochorionic diamniotic twin pregnancy complicated by selective fetal growth restriction. Ultrasound Obstet Gynecol. 2019; 53: 200–7.

232 Townsend, R, Duffy, JMN, Sileo, F, et al. International Collaboration to Harmonise Outcomes for Selective Fetal Growth Restriction (CHOOSE-FGR). Core outcome set for studies investigating management of selective fetal growth restriction in twins. Ultrasound Obstet Gynecol. 2020; 55: 652–60.

233 Khairudin, D, Khalil, A. Monochorionic monoamniotic twin pregnancies. Best Pract Res Clin Obstet Gynaecol. 2022; 84: 96–103.

234 Saccone, G, Khalil, A, Thilaganathan, B, et al. Weight discordance and perinatal mortality in monoamniotic twin pregnancy: analysis of MONOMONO, NorSTAMP and STORK multiple-pregnancy cohorts. Ultrasound Obstet Gynecol. 2020; 55: 332–8.

235 MONOMONO Working Group. Inpatient vs outpatient management and timing of delivery of uncomplicated monochorionic monoamniotic twin pregnancy: the MONOMONO study. Ultrasound Obstet Gynecol. 2019; 53: 175–83.

236 Madsen, C, Sogaard, K, Zingenberg, H, et al. Outcomes of monoamniotic twin pregnancies managed primarily in outpatient care-a Danish multi-center study. Acta Obstet Gynecol Scand. 2019; 98: 479–86.

237 Quinn, KH, Cao, CT, Lacoursiere, DY, Schrimmer, D. Monoamniotic twin pregnancy: continuous inpatient electronic fetal monitoring-an impossible goal? Am J Obstet Gynecol. 2011; 204: 161e1–6.

238 Committee opinion no. 719 summary: multifetal pregnancy reduction. Obstet Gynecol. 2017; 130: 670–1.

239 Beriwal, S, Impey, L, Ioannou, C. Multifetal pregnancy reduction and selective termination. Obstet Gynecol. 2020; 22: 284–92.

240 Dodd, J, Crowther, C. Multifetal pregnancy reduction of triplet and higher-order multiple pregnancies to twins. Fertil Steril. 2004; 81: 1420–2.

241 Gaerty, K, Greer, RM, Kumar, S. Systematic review and metaanalysis of perinatal outcomes after radiofrequency ablation and bipolar cord

occlusion in monochorionic pregnancies. Am J Obstet Gynecol. 2015; 213: 637–43.

242 Anthoulakis, C, Dagklis, T, Mamopoulos, A, Athanasiadis, A. Risks of miscarriage or preterm delivery in trichorionic and dichorionic triplet pregnancies with embryo reduction versus expectant management: a systematic review and meta-analysis. Hum Reprod. 2017; 32: 1351–9.

243 Chaveeva, P, Kosinski, P, Puglia, D, Poon, LC, Nicolaides, KH. Trichorionic and dichorionic triplet pregnancies at 10–14 weeks: outcome after embryo reduction compared to expectant management. Fetal Diagn Ther. 2013; 34: 199–205.

244 Morlando, M, Ferrara, L, d'Antonio, F, et al. Dichorionic triplet pregnancies: risk of miscarriage and severe preterm delivery with fetal reduction versus expectant management. Outcomes of a cohort study and systematic review. BJOG. 2015; 122: 1053–60.

245 Kumar, S, Paramasivam, G, Zhang, E, et al. Perinatal- and procedure-related outcomes following radiofrequency ablation in monochorionic pregnancy. Am J Obstet Gynecol. 2014; 210: 454.e1–6.

246 Chaveeva, P, Peeva, G, Pugliese, SG, Shterev, A, Nicolaides, KH. Intrafetal laser ablation for embryo reduction from dichorionic triplets to dichorionic twins. Ultrasound Obstet Gynecol. 2017; 50: 632–4.

247 Curado, J, d'antonio, F, Papageorghiou, AT, et al. Perinatal mortality and morbidity in triplet pregnancy according to chorionicity: systematic review and meta-analysis. Ultrasound Obstet Gynecol. 2019; 54: 589–95.

248 Antsaklis, A, Anastasakis, E. Selective reduction in twins and multiple pregnancies. J Perinat Med. 2011; 39: 15–21.

249 Zipori, Y, Haas, J, Berger, H, Barzilay, E. Multifetal pregnancy reduction of triplets to twins compared with non-reduced triplets: a meta-analysis. Reprod Biomed Online. 2017; 35: 296–304.

250 Schreiner-Engel, P, Walther, VN, Mindes, J, Lynch, L, Berkowitz, RL. First-trimester multifetal pregnancy reduction: acute and persistent psychologic reactions. Am J Obstet Gynecol. 1995; 172: 541–7.

251 Stone, J, Ferrara, L, Kamrath, J, et al. Contemporary outcomes with the latest 1000 cases of multifetal pregnancy reduction (MPR). Am J Obstet Gynecol. 2008; 199: 406.e1–4.

252 Bigelow, CA, Factor, SH, Moshier, E, et al. Timing of and outcomes after selective termination of anomalous fetuses in dichorionic twin pregnancies. Prenat Diagn. 2014; 34: 1320–5.

253 Sorrenti, S, di Mascio, D, Khalil, A, et al. Pregnancy and perinatal outcomes of early vs late selective termination in dichorionic twin pregnancy:

systematic review and meta-analysis. Ultrasound Obstet Gynecol. 2023; 61(5): 552–8. http://dx.doi.org/10.1002/uog.26126.

254 Ting, YH, Poon, LCY, Tse, WT, et al. Outcome of radiofrequency ablation for selective fetal reduction before vs at or after 16 gestational weeks in complicated monochorionic pregnancy. Ultrasound Obstet Gynecol. 2021; 58: 214–20.

255 van den Bos, EM, van Klink, JM, Middeldorp, JM, et al. Perinatal outcome after selective feticide in monochorionic twin pregnancies. Ultrasound Obstet Gynecol. 2013; 41: 653–8.

256 Hillman, S, Morris, R, Kilby, M. Single twin demise: consequence for survivors. Semin Fetal Neonat Med. 2010; 15: 319–26.

257 Mcpherson, JA, Odibo, AO, Shanks, AL, et al. Impact of chorionicity on risk and timing of intrauterine fetal demise in twin pregnancies. Am J Obstet Gynecol. 2012; 207: 190.e1–6.

258 Gurney, L, Morris, RK, Gibson, J, Kilby, M. Fetal demise in twins: single and double fetal loss. In: Twin and Higher-Order Pregnancies. London: Springer, 2021, 205–27.

259 Healy, EF, Khalil, A. Single intrauterine death in twin pregnancy: evidenced-based counselling and management. Best Pract Res Clin Obstet Gynaecol. 2022; 84: 205–17.

260 Ward, PL, Reidy, KL, Palma-Dias, R, Doyle, LW, Umstad, MP. Single intrauterine death in twins: the importance of fetal order. Twin Res Hum Genet. 2018; 21: 556–62.

261 Brassard, M, Fouron, JC, Leduc, L, Grignon, A, Proulx, F. Prognostic markers in twin pregnancies with an acardiac fetus. Obstet Gynecol. 1999; 94: 409–14.

262 Mone, F, Devaseelan, P, Ong, S. Intervention versus a conservative approach in the management of TRAP sequence: a systematic review. J Perinat Med. 2016; 44: 619–29.

263 Gabby, LC, Chon, AC, Korst, LM, Llanes, A, Chmait, RH. Risk factors for co-twin fetal demise following radiofrequency ablation in multifetal monochorionic gestations. Fetal Diagn Ther. 2020; 47(11): 1–7.

264 Wang, H, Zhou, Q, Wang, X, et al. Influence of indications on perinatal outcomes after radio frequency ablation in complicated monochorionic pregnancies: a retrospective cohort study. BMC Pregnancy Childbirth. 2021; 21: 41.

265 Rahimi-Sharbaf, F, Ghaemi, M, Nassr, AA, Shamshirsaz, AA, Shirazi, M. Radiofrequency ablation for selective fetal reduction in complicated mono-chorionic twins; comparing the outcomes according to the indications. BMC Pregnancy Childbirth. 2021; 21: 189.

266 Sun, L, Zou, G, Yang, Y, Zhou, F, Tao, D. Risk factors for fetal death after radiofrequency ablation for complicated monochorionic twin pregnancies. Prenat Diagn. 2018; 38: 499–503.

267 Peng, R, Xie, HN, Lin, MF, et al. Clinical outcomes after selective fetal reduction of complicated monochorionic twins with radiofrequency ablation and bipolar cord coagulation. Gynecol Obstet Invest. 2016; 81: 552–8.

268 Has, R, Kalelioglu, I, Corbacioglu Esmer, A, et al. Bipolar cord coagulation in the management of complicated monochorionic twin pregnancies. Fetal Diagn Ther. 2014; 36: 190–5.

269 Donepudi, R, Hessami, K, Nassr, AA, et al. Selective reduction in complicated monochorionic pregnancies: a systematic review and meta-analysis of different techniques. Am J Obstet Gynecol. 2022; 226: 646–55.

270 Meng, X, Yuan, P, Gong, L, et al. Forty-five consecutive cases of complicated monochorionic multiple pregnancy treated with microwave ablation: a single-center experience. Prenat Diagn. 2019; 39: 293–8.

271 Xie, J, Cheng, Z, Wu, T, Wei, Y, Wang, X. Microwave ablation versus radiofrequency ablation for the treatment of severe complicated monochorionic pregnancies in China: protocol for a pilot randomised controlled trial. BMJ Open. 2020; 10: e034995.

272 Tavares de Sousa, M, Glosemeyer, P, Diemert, A, Bamberg, C, Hecher, K. First-trimester intervention in twin reversed arterial perfusion sequence. Ultrasound Obstet Gynecol. 2019; 55: 47–9.

273 Weber, EC, Recker, F, Gottschalk, I, et al. Outcome of monochorionic monoamniotic twin reversed arterial perfusion sequence diagnosed in the first trimester. Fetal Diagn Ther. 2021; 48: 778–84.

274 TRAP Intervention Study:: early versus late intervention for twin reversed arterial perfusion sequence. clinicaltrials.gov. 2017. Report No.: NCT02621645. https://clinicaltrials.gov/ct2/show/NCT02621645 (accessed 15 September 2024).

275 Denbow, M, Fogliani, R, Kyle, P, et al. Haematological indices at fetal blood sampling in monochorionic pregnancies complicated by feto-fetal transfusion syndrome. Prenat Diagn. 1998; 18: 941–6.

276 Paek, B, Dorn, M, Walker, M. Atypical twin-to-twin transfusion syndrome: prevalence in a population undergoing fetoscopic laser ablation of communicating placental vessels. Am J Obstet Gynecol. 2016; 215: e1–5.

277 Solorio, C, Guenther, JS, Chon, AH, et al. Twin–twin transfusion syndrome and the definition of recipient polyhydramnios. Am J Obstet Gynecol. 2021; 225: e1–8.

278 Khalil, A. Modified diagnostic criteria for twin-to-twin transfusion syndrome prior to 18 weeks' gestation: time to change? Ultrasound Obstet Gynecol. 2021; 49: 804–5.

279 Khalil, A, Liu, B. Controversies in the management of twin pregnancy. Ultrasound Obstet Gynecol. 2021; 57: 888–902.

280 Lopriore, E, Sueters, M, Middeldorp, JM, et al. Neonatal outcome in twin-to-twin transfusion syndrome treated with fetoscopic laser occlusion of vascular anastomoses. J Pediatr. 2005; 147: 597–602.

281 Roberts, D, Neilson, JP, Kilby, MD, Gates, S. Interventions for the treatment of twin–twin transfusion syndrome. Cochrane Database Syst Rev. 2014; (1): CD002073.

282 Senat, MV, Deprest, J, Boulvain, M, et al. Endoscopic laser surgery versus serial amnioreduction for severe twin-to-twin transfusion syndrome. N Engl J Med. 2004; 351: 136–44.

283 Crombleholme, TM, Shera, D, Lee, H, et al. A prospective, randomized, multicenter trial of amnioreduction vs selective fetoscopic laser photocoagulation for the treatment of severe twin–twin transfusion syndrome. Am J Obstet Gynecol. 2007; 197: 396.e1–9.

284 Khalil, A, Cooper, E, Townsend, R, Thilaganathan, B. Evolution of stage 1 twin-to-twin transfusion syndrome (TTTS): systematic review and meta-analysis. Twin Res Hum Genet. 2016; 19: 207–16.

285 di Mascio, D, Khalil, A, d'Amico, A, et al. Outcome of twin–twin transfusion syndrome according to Quintero stage of disease: systematic review and meta-analysis. Ultrasound Obstet Gynecol. 2020; 56: 811–20.

286 Stirnemann, J, Slaghekke, F, Khalek, N, et al. Intrauterine fetoscopic laser surgery versus expectant management in stage 1 twin-to-twin transfusion syndrome: an international randomized trial. Am J Obstet Gynecol. 2021; 224: 528.e1–e12.

287 Wohlmuth, C, Gardiner, HM. Twin–twin transfusion syndrome: don't rely on fluids and bladders to catch it early. Ultrasound Obstet Gynecol. 2022; 59: 7–10.

288 Nassr, AA, Hessami, K, Espinoza, J, et al. Gestational age and Quintero staging as predictors of single fetal demise in twin–twin transfusion syndrome after fetoscopic laser photocoagulation: a systematic review and meta-analysis. AJOG Glob Rep. 2022; 2(3): 100055.

289 Murgano, D, Khalil, A, Prefumo, F, et al. Outcome of twin-to-twin transfusion syndrome in monochorionic monoamniotic twin pregnancy: systematic review and meta-analysis. Ultrasound Obstet Gynecol. 2020; 55: 310–17.

290 Lopriore, E, Middeldorp, JM, Oepkes, D, et al. Residual anastomoses after fetoscopic laser surgery in twin-to-twin transfusion syndrome: frequency, associated risks and outcome. Placenta. 2007; 28: 204–8.

291 Robyr, R, Lewi, L, Salomon, LJ, et al. Prevalence and management of late fetal complications following successful selective laser coagulation of chorionic plate anastomoses in twin-to-twin transfusion syndrome. Am J Obstet Gynecol. 2006; 194: 796–803.

292 Slaghekke, F, Lopriore, E, Lewi, L, et al. Fetoscopic laser coagulation of the vascular equator versus selective coagulation for twin-to-twin transfusion syndrome: an open-label randomised controlled trial. Lancet. 2014; 383: 2144–51.

293 van Klink, JM, Slaghekke, F, Balestriero, MA, et al. Neurodevelopmental outcome at 2 years in twin–twin transfusion syndrome survivors randomized for the Solomon trial. Am J Obstet Gynecol. 2016; 214: 113.e1–7.

294 Dhillon, RK, Hillman, SC, Pounds, R, Morris, RK, Kilby, MD. Comparison of Solomon technique against selective laser ablation for twin–twin transfusion syndrome: a systematic review. Ultrasound Obstet Gynecol. 2015; 46: 526–31.

295 Kanazawa, S, Ozawa, K, Muromoto, J, et al. Risk profiling of the Solomon technique versus selective technique of fetoscopic laser surgery for twin–twin transfusion syndrome. Twin Res Hum Genet. 2021; 24: 42–8.

296 Knijnenburg, PJC, Lopriore, E, Ge, Y, et al. Placental abruption after fetoscopic laser surgery in twin–twin transfusion syndrome: the role of the solomon technique. Fetal Diagn Ther. 2021; 48: 660–66.

297 Morris, RK, Selman, TJ, Harbidge, A, Martin, WI, Kilby, MD. Fetoscopic laser coagulation for severe twin-to-twin transfusion syndrome: factors influencing perinatal outcome, learning curve of the procedure and lessons for new centres. BJOG. 2010; 117: 1350–7.

298 Aboudiab, MS, Chon, AH, Korst, LM, et al. Management of twin–twin transfusion syndrome with an extremely short cervix. J Obstet Gynaecol. 2018; 38: 359–62.

299 Malshe, A, Snowise, S, Mann, LK, et al. Preterm delivery after fetoscopic laser surgery for twin–twin transfusion syndrome: etiology and risk factors. Ultrasound Obstet Gynecol. 2017; 49: 612–16.

300 Papanna, R, Habli, M, Baschat, AA, et al. Cerclage for cervical shortening at fetoscopic laser photocoagulation in twin–twin transfusion syndrome. Am J Obstet Gynecol. 2012; 206: 425 e1–7.

301 Buskmiller, C, Bergh, EP, Brock, C, et al. Interventions to prevent preterm delivery in women with short cervix before fetoscopic laser surgery for

twin–twin transfusion syndrome. Ultrasound Obstet Gynecol. 2022; 59: 169–76.

302 Tollenaar, LSA, Loprior, E, Oepkes, D, et al. Twin anemia polycythemia sequence: knowledge and insights after 15 years of research. Maternal Fetal Medicine 2021; 3(1): 33–41.

303 Tollenaar, LSA, Lopriore, E, Middeldorp, JM, et al. Improved prediction of twin anemia–polycythemia sequence by delta middle cerebral artery peak systolic velocity: new antenatal classification system. Ultrasound Obstet Gynecol. 2019; 53: 788–93.

304 Tavares de Sousa, M, Fonseca, A, Hecher, K. Role of fetal intertwin difference in middle cerebral artery peak systolic velocity in predicting neonatal twin anemia–polycythemia sequence. Ultrasound Obstet Gynecol. 2019; 53: 794–7.

305 Khalil, A, Gordijn, S, Ganzevoort, W, et al. Consensus diagnostic criteria and monitoring of twin anemia–polycythemia sequence: Delphi procedure. Ultrasound Obstet Gynecol. 2020; 56: 388–94.

306 Baschat, AA, Miller, JL. Pathophysiology, diagnosis, and management of twin anemia polycythemia sequence in monochorionic multiple gestations. Best Pract Res Clin Obstet Gynaecol. 2022; 84: 115-26.

307 Denbow, ML, Eckersley, R, Welsh, AW, et al. Ex vivo delineation of placental angioarchitecture with the microbubble contrast agent levovist. Am J Obstet Gynecol. 2000; 182: 966–71.

308 Slaghekke, F, Kist, WJ, Oepkes, D, et al. Twin anemia–polycythemia sequence: diagnostic criteria, classification, perinatal management and outcome. Fetal Diagn Ther. 2010; 27: 181–90.

309 Bahtiyar, MO, Ekmekci, E, Demirel, E, Irani, RA, Copel, JA. In utero partial exchange transfusion combined with in utero blood transfusion for prenatal management of twin anemia–polycythemia sequence. Fetal Diagn Ther. 2019; 45: 28–35.

310 Herway, C, Johnson, A, Moise, K, Moise, K J. Fetal intraperitoneal transfusion for iatrogenic twin anemia–polycythemia sequence after laser therapy. Ultrasound Obstet Gynecol. 2009; 33: 592–4.

311 Tollenaar, LSA, Slaghekke, F, Lewi, L, et al. Treatment and outcome of 370 cases with spontaneous or post-laser twin anemia–polycythemia sequence managed in 17 fetal therapy centers. Ultrasound Obstet Gynecol. 2020; 56: 378–87.

312 Gibson, JL, Castleman, JS, Meher, S, Kilby, MD. Updated guidance for the management of twin and triplet pregnancies from the National Institute for Health and Care Excellence guidance, UK: what's new that may improve perinatal outcomes? Acta Obstet Gynecol Scand. 2020; 99: 147–52.

313 Giorgione, V, d'Antonio, F, Manji, A, Reed, K, Khalil, A. Perinatal outcome of pregnancy complicated by twin anemia–polycythemia sequence: systematic review and meta-analysis. Ultrasound Obstet Gynecol. 2021; 58: 813–23.

314 Leiden University Medical Center. The TAPS Trial – fetoscopic laser surgery for twin anemia polycythemia sequence. clinicaltrials.gov. 2020. Report No.: NCT04432168. https://clinicaltrials.gov/ct2/show/ NCT04432168 (accessed 15 September 2024).

315 Tollenaar, LSA, Lopriore, E, Slaghekke, F, et al. High risk of long-term neurodevelopmental impairment in donor twins with spontaneous twin anemia–polycythemia sequence. Ultrasound Obstet Gynecol. 2020; 55: 39–46.

316 Greco, PS, Pitts, D, Weadock, WJ, et al. Conjoined twins: an obstetrician's guide to prenatal care and delivery management. J Perinatol. 202; 41: 2424–31.

317 Afzal, AR, Montero, FJ. Conjoined Twins. Treasure Island, FL: StatPearls Publishing, 2022.

318 Sager, EC, Thomas, A, Sundgren, NC. Conjoined twins: pre-birth management, changes to NRP, and transport. Semin Perinatol. 2018; 42: 321–8.

319 Martin, JA, Hamilton, BE, Sutton, PD, et al. National Vital Statistics Report 2010. Natl Vital Stat Rep. 2010; 59(1): 3–71.

320 Stoenescu, A, Friedl, WPT, de-Gregorio, N, et al. A single-center cohort study on 1663 twin births from two decades: a descriptive statistics and general trends. Gynecol Obstet (Sunnyvale). 2020; 10: 520.

321 Dodd, JM, Deussen, AR, Grivell, RM, Crowther, CA. Elective birth at 37 weeks' gestation for women with an uncomplicated twin pregnancy. Cochrane Database Syst Rev. 2014; (2): CD003582.

322 Dodd, JM, Crowther, CA, Haslam, RR, Robinson, JS. Elective birth at 37 weeks of gestation versus standard care for women with an uncomplicated twin pregnancy at term: the Twins Timing of Birth Randomised Trial. BJOG. 2012; 119: 964–73.

323 Cheong-See, F, Schuit, E, Arroyo-Manzano, D, et al. Prospective risk of stillbirth and neonatal complications in twin pregnancies: systematic review and meta-analysis. BMJ. 2016; 354: i4353.

324 Bibbo, C, Robinson, JN. Management of twins: vaginal or cesarean delivery? Clin Obstet Gynecol. 2015; 58: 294–308.

325 Lee, YM. Delivery of twins. Semin Perinatol. 2012; 36: 195–200.

326 The Royal Australian and New Zealand College of Obstericians and Gynaecologists (RANZCOG). Management of Breech Presentation. Best practice statement. Melbourne, RANZCOG, 2021.

327 Hannah, ME, Hannah, WJ, Hewson, SA, et al. Planned cesarean section versus planned vaginal birth for breech presentation at term: a randomised multicentre trial. Lancet. 2000; 356: 1375–83.

328 Hofmeyr, GJ, Hannah, M, Lawrie, TA. Planned cesarean section for term breech delivery. Cochrane Database Syst Rev. 2015; (7): CD000166.

329 Hogle, KL, Hutton, EK, McBrien, KA, Barrett, JF, Hannah, ME. Cesarean delivery for twins: a systematic review and meta-analysis. Am J Obstet Gynecol. 2003; 188: 220–7.

330 Steins Bisschop, CN, Vogelvang, TE, May, AM, Schuitemaker, NW. Mode of delivery in non-cephalic presenting twins: a systematic review. Arch Gynecol Obstet. 2012; 286: 237–47.

331 Korb, D, Goffinet, F, Bretelle, F, et al. First twin in breech presentation and neonatal mortality and morbidity according to planned mode of delivery. Obstet Gynecol. 2020; 135: 1015–23.

332 Felder, L, McCurdy, R, Berghella, V. External cephalic version of the non-cephalic presenting twin: a systematic review. J Matern Fetal Neonatal Med. 2022; 35: 1712–18.

333 Impey, LWM, Murphy, DJ, Griffiths, M, Penna, LK, on behalf of the Royal College of Obstetricians and Gynaecologists. Management of breech presentation. BJOG. 2017; 124: e151–77.

334 Rossi, AC, Mullin, PM, Chmait, RH. Neonatal outcomes of twins according to birth order, presentation and mode of delivery: a systematic review and meta-analysis. BJOG. 2011; 118: 523–32.

335 Barrett, JF, Hannah, ME, Hutton, EK, et al. Twin Birth Study Collaborative Group. A randomized trial of planned cesarean or vaginal delivery for twin pregnancy. N Engl J Med. 2013; 369: 1295–305.

336 Asztalos, EV, Hannah, ME, Hutton, EK, et al. Twin birth study: 2 year neurodevelopmental follow-up of the randomized trial of planned caesarean or planned vaginal delivery for twin pregnancy. Am J Obstet Gynecol 2016; 214(3): 371.e1–19.

337 Vogel, JP, Holloway, E, Cuesta, C, et al. Outcomes of non-vertex second twins, following vertex vaginal delivery of first twin: a secondary analysis of the WHO Global Survey on maternal and perinatal health. BMC Pregnancy Childbirth. 2014; 14: 55.

338 Cohen, R, Kashani Ligumsky, L, Lopian, M, et al. Is vaginal delivery of a breech second twin safe? A comparison between delivery of vertex and non-vertex second twins. J Matern Fetal Neonatal Med. 2022; 35: 8852–5.

339 Schmitz, T, Korb, D, Battie, C, et al. Neonatal morbidity associated with vaginal delivery of noncephalic second twins. Am J Obstet Gynecol. 2018; 218: 449.e1–449.e13.

340 Cahill, A, Stamilio, D, Pare, E, Peipert, J, Macones, G. Vaginal birth after cesarean (VBAC) in twin pregnancies: Is it safe? Am J Obstet Gynaecol. 2004; 191(6), suppl. S183. https://doi.org/10.1016/j.ajog.2004.10.557.

341 Myles, T. Vaginal birth of twins after a previous cesarean section. J Matern Fetal Med. 2001; 10: 171–4.

342 Hochler, H, Tevet, A, Barg, M, et al. Trial of labor of vertex-nonvertex twins following a previous cesarean delivery. Am J Obstet Gynecol MFM. 2022; 4: 100640.

343 Baradaran, K. Risk of uterine rupture with vaginal birth after cesarean in twin gestations. Obstet Gynecol Int. 2021; 2021: 6693142.

344 Gerten, KA, Coonrod, DV, Bay, RC, Chambliss, LR. Cesarean delivery and respiratory distress syndrome: does labor make a difference? Am J Obstet Gynecol. 2005; 193(3 Pt 2): 1061–4.

345 Vidic, Z, Blickstein, I, Štucin Gantar, I, Verdenik, I, Tul, N. Timing of elective cesarean section and neonatal morbidity: a population-based study. J Matern Fetal Neonatal Med. 2016; 29: 2461–3.

346 Bricelj, K, Tul, N, Lasic, M, et al. Respiratory morbidity in twins by birth order, gestational age and mode of delivery. J Perinat Med. 2016; 44: 899–902.

347 Royal College of Obstetricians and Gynecologists (RCOG). Antenatal Corticosteroids to Reduce Neonatal Morbidity and Mortality. Green-top guideline no. 74. London: RCOG, 2022.

348 Negrini, R, da Silva Ferreira, RD, Guimarães, DZ. Value-based care in obstetrics: comparison between vaginal birth and cesarean section. BMC Pregnancy Childbirth. 2021; 21: 333.

349 Mol, BW, Bergenhenegouwen, L, Ensing, S, Ravelli, AC, Kok, M. The impact of mode of delivery on the outcome in very preterm twins. J Matern Fetal Neonatal Med. 2020; 33: 2089–95.

350 Sentilhes, L, Lorthe, E, Marchand-Martin, L, et al. Planned mode of delivery of preterm twins and neonatal and 2-year outcomes. Obstet Gynecol. 2019; 133: 71–80.

351 Yang, Q, Wen, SW, Chen, Y, et al. Neonatal death and morbidity in vertex-nonvertex second twins according to mode of delivery and birth weight. Am J Obstet Gynecol. 2005; 192: 840–7.

352 Dagenais, C, Lewis-Mikhael, AM, Grabovac, M, Mukerji, A, McDonald, SD. What is the safest mode of delivery for extremely preterm cephalic/non-cephalic twin pairs? A systematic review and meta-analyses. BMC Pregnancy Childbirth. 2017; 17: 397.

353 Hiersch, L, Shah, PS, Mcdonald, SD, Barrett, J, Melamed, N. 946: Mode of delivery and the risk of adverse outcomes in preterm twins <28 weeks. Am J Obstet Gynecol. 2020; 222: S586–7.

354 Tucker Edmonds, B, McKenzie, F, Macheras, M, Srinivas, SK, Lorch, SA. Morbidity and mortality associated with mode of delivery for breech periviable deliveries. Am J Obstet Gynecol. 2015; 213: 70.e1–12.

355 McDonald, SD, Narvey, M, Ehman, W, Jain, V, Cassell, K. Guideline No. 424: Umbilical cord management in preterm and term infants. J Obstet Gynaecol Can. 2022; 44: 313–322.e1.

356 Grabovac, M, Beltempo, M, Lodha, A, et al. Impact of deferred cord clamping on mortality and severe neurologic injury in twins born at <30 weeks of gestation. J Pediatr. 2021; 238: 118–23.e3.

357 Liu, LY, Yee, LM. Delayed cord clamping in preterm dichorionic twin gestations. J Matern Fetal Neonatal Med. 2019; 26: 1–5.

358 Ruangkit, C, Bumrungphuet, S, Panburana, P, Khositseth, A, Nuntnarumit, P. A randomized controlled trial of immediate versus delayed umbilical cord clamping in multiple-birth infants born preterm. Neonatology. 2019; 115: 156–63.

359 Acker, D, Lieberman, M, Holbrook, RH, et al. Delivery of the second twin. Obstet Gynecol. 1982; 59: 710–11.

360 Chervenak, FA, Johnson, RE, Berkowitz, RL, Hobbins, JC. Intrapartum external version of the second twin. Obstet Gynecol.1983; 62: 160–5.

361 Chauhan, SP, Roberts, WE, McLaren, RA, et al. Delivery of the nonvertex second twin: breech extraction versus external cephalic version. Am J Obstet Gynecol. 1995; 173: 1015–20.

362 Webster, SN, Loughney, AD. Internal podalic version with breech extraction. Obstet Gynecol. 2011; 13: 7–14.

363 Stein, W, Misselwitz, B, Schmidt, S. Twin-to-twin delivery time interval: influencing factors and effect on short-term outcome of the second twin. Acta Obstet Gynecol Scand. 2008; 87: 346–53.

364 Lindroos, L, Elfvin, A, Ladfors, L, Wennerholm, UB. The effect of twin-to-twin delivery time intervals on neonatal outcome for second twins. BMC Pregnancy Childbirth. 2018; 18: 36.

365 Leung, TY, Tam, WH, Leung, TN, Lok, IH, Lau, TK. Effect of twin-to-twin delivery interval on umbilical cord blood gas in the second twins. BJOG. 2002; 109: 63–7.

366 Cukierman, R, Heland, S, Palmer, K, et al. Inter-twin delivery interval, short-term perinatal outcomes and risk of cesarean for the second twin. Aust N Z J Obstet Gynaecol. 2019; 59: 375–9.

367 McGrail, CD, Bryant, DR. Intertwin time interval: how it affects the immediate neonatal outcome of the second twin. Am J Obstet Gynecol. 2005; 192: 1420–2.

368 Wenze, SJ, Battle, CL, Tezanos, KM. Raising multiples: mental health of mothers and fathers in early parenthood. Arch Womens Ment Health. 2015; 18: 163–76.

369 Robertson, E, Celasun, N, Stewart, DE. Risk factors for postpartum depression. In: Stewart, DE, Robertson, E, Dennis, CL, Grace, SL, Wallington, T (eds.), Postpartum Depression: Literature Review of Risk Factors and Interventions. Toronto: Toronto Public Health, 2003.

370 Smith, LK, Manktelow, BN, Draper, ED, et al. Trends in the incidence and mortality of multiple births by socioeconomic deprivation and maternal age in England: population-based cohort study. BMJ Open. 2014; 4: e004514.

371 The Fetal Medicine Foundation. Protocol for Ultrasound Scans. https://fetalmedicine.org/education/fetal-abnormalities/multiple-pregnancies/protocol-for-ultrasound-scans (accessed 16 September 2024).

Cambridge Elements⩵

High-Risk Pregnancy: Management Options

Professor David James

Emeritus Professor, University of Nottingham, UK

David James was Professor of Fetomaternal Medicine at the University of Nottingham from 1992–2009. The post involved clinical service, especially the management of high-risk pregnancies, guideline development, research and teaching and NHS management. From 2009–14 he was Clinical Director of Women's Health at the National Centre for Clinical Excellence for Women's and Children's Health. He was also Clinical Lead for the RCOG/RCM/ eLfH eFM E-Learning Project. He is a recognised authority on the management of problem/ complicated pregnancies with over 200 peer-reviewed publications. He has published 16 books, the best-known being *High-Risk Pregnancy: Management Options*.

Professor Philip Steer

Emeritus Professor, Imperial College, London, UK

Philip Steer is Emeritus Professor of Obstetrics at Imperial College London, having been appointed Professor in 1989. He was a consultant obstetrician for 35 years. He was Editor-in-Chief of *BJOG – An International Journal of Obstetrics and Gynaecology* – from 2005–2012, and is now Editor Emeritus. He has published more than 150 peer-reviewed research papers, 109 reviews and editorials and 66 book chapters/books, the best known and most successful being *High-Risk Pregnancy: Management Options*. The fifth edition was published in 2018. He has been President of the British Association of Perinatal Medicine and President of the Section of Obstetrics and Gynaecology of the Royal Society of Medicine. He is an honorary fellow of the College of Obstetricians and Gynaecologists of South Africa, and of the American Gynecological & Obstetrical Society.

Professor Carl Weiner

Creighton University School of Medicine, Phoenix, AZ, USA

Carl Weiner is presently Head of Maternal Fetal Medicine for the CommonSpirit Health System, Arizona, Director of Maternal Fetal Medicine, Dignity St Joseph's Hospital, Professor, Obstetrics and Gynecology, Creighton School of Medicine, Phoenix, and Professor, College of Health Solutions, Arizona State University. He is the former Krantz Professor and Chair of Obstetrics and Gynecology, Division Head Maternal Fetal Medicine and Professor Molecular and Integrative Physiology at the University of Kansas School of Medicine, Kansas City, KS and the Crenshaw Professor and Chair of Obstetrics, Gynecology and Reproductive Biology, Division Head Maternal Fetal Medicine, and Professor of Physiology at the University of Maryland School of Medicine, Baltimore. Dr Weiner has published more than 265 peer-reviewed research articles and authored/edited 18 textbooks including *High-Risk Pregnancy: Management Options*. His research was extramurally funded for more than 30 years without interruption.

Professor Stephen Robson

Newcastle University, UK

Stephen C. Robson is Emeritus Professor of Fetal Medicine for the Population and Health Sciences Institute at The Medical School, Newcastle University. He is also a Consultant in Fetal Medicine for Newcastle upon Tyne Hospitals NHS Foundation Trust. He has published over 400 peer-reviewed articles and edited several; books, the highly successful being *High Risk Pregnancy: Management Options*. The fifth edition was published in 2018. He has been President of the British Maternal and Fetal Medicine.

About the Series

Most pregnancies are uncomplicated. However, for some ('high-risk' pregnancies) an adverse outcome for the mother and/or the baby is more likely. Each Element in the series covers a specific high-risk problem/condition in pregnancy. The risks of the condition will be listed followed by an evidence-based review of the management options. Once the series is complete, the Elements will be collated and printed in a sixth edition of *High-Risk Pregnancy: Management Options*.

Cambridge Elements ≡

High-Risk Pregnancy: Management Options

Elements in the Series

Fetal Compromise in Labor
Mark I. Evans, Lawrence D. Devoe and Philip J. Steer

Spontaneous Preterm Labour and Birth (Including Preterm Pre-labour Rupture of Membranes)
Natasha L. Hezelgrave and Andrew H. Shennan

Multiple Pregnancy
Jack Hamer, Jennifer Tamblyn, James Castleman and R. Katie Morris

A full series listing is available at: www.cambridge.org/EHRP

Printed in the United States
by Baker & Taylor Publisher Services